Host-Parasite Relationships in Systemic Mycoses
Part I: Methodology, Pathology and Immunology

Contributions to Microbiology and Immunology

Vol. 3

Series Editors
J. Lindenmann and H. Ramseier, Zürich

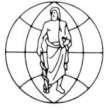

S. Karger · Basel · München · Paris · London · New York · Sydney

Proceedings of the 21st Annual OHOLO Biological Conference,
Ma'alot, Israel, March 28–31, 1976

Host-Parasite Relationships in Systemic Mycoses

Part I: Methodology, Pathology and Immunology

Volume Editors
A.M. Beemer; A. Ben-David; M.A. Klingberg, and E.S. Kuttin, Ness-Ziona

Technical Editor: *Myra Kaye*

41 figures and 26 tables, 1977

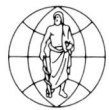

S. Karger · Basel · München · Paris · London · New York · Sydney

Contributions to Microbiology and Immunology

Vol. 1: Staphylococci and Staphylococcal Infections. Recent Progress. Proceedings of the 2nd International Symposium, Warszawa 1971. Editor: J. Jeljaszewicz (Warszawa); Associated Editor: W. Hryniewicz (Warszawa).
XII + 658 p., 260 fig., 333 tab., 1973. ISBN 3-8055-1634-7

Vol. 2: Yersinia, Pasteurella and Francisella. Proceedings of the International Symposium, Malmö 1972.
Series Editor: A. Grumbach (Zürich); Volume Editor: S. Winblad (Malmö).
XIV + 242 p., 55 fig., 89 tab., 1973. ISBN 3-8055-1636-3

Cataloging in Publication

Oholo Biological Conference, 21st, Ma'alot, Israel, 1976
Host-parasite relationships in systemic mycoses: proceedings of the
21st annual OHOLO Biological Conference, Ma'alot, Israel, March 28–31, 1976
Volume editors, A.M. Beemer . . . (et al.). – Basel; New York; Karger, 1977.
(Contributions to microbiology and immunology; v. 3–4)
Contents: pt. 1. Methodology, pathology and immunology. – pt. 2. Specific diseases and therapy. Organized and sponsored by the Israel Institute for Biological Research
1. Mycoses – congresses 2. Symbiosis – congresses I. Beemer, A.M., ed.
II. Israel Institute for Biological Research III. Title IV. Series
W1 C0778UK v. 3–4/ WC 450 038 1976h
ISBN 3-8055-2443-9

All rights reserved.
No part of this publication may be translated into other languages, reproduced or utilized in any form or by any means, electronic or mechanical, including photocopying, recording, microcopying, or by any information storage and retrieval system, without permission in writing from the publisher.

© Copyright 1977 by S. Karger AG, 4011 Basel (Switzerland), Arnold-Böcklin-Strasse 25
ISBN 3-8055-2443-9

Contents

Host-Parasite Relationships in Systemic Mycoses
Part I: Methodology, Pathology and Immunology

Part II of the Proceedings of the 21st Annual OHOLO Biological Conference, Ma'alot, Israel 1976, is published as Vol. 4 of 'Contributions to Microbiology and Immunology'. For table of contents see page VI of this volume.

Conference Organizing Committee VII
Acknowledgments VIII
List of Participants IX
Preface XII

Ben-David, A. (Ness-Ziona): Introductory Remarks 1
Ajello, L. (Atlanta, Ga.): Systemic Mycoses in Modern Medicine 2
Ajello, L. (Atlanta, Ga.): Medically Important Infectious Fungi 7
Kaplan, W. (Atlanta, Ga.): Diagnosis of Systemic Mycoses 20
Louria, D.B. (Newark, N.J.): Experimental Infections with Fungi and Yeasts 31
Staib, F.; Mishra, S.K.; Grosse, G., and Abel, R. (Berlin): Pathogenesis and Therapy of Cryptococcosis in Animal Experiments 48
Shahar, A.; Kletter, Y., and Aronson, M. (Tel-Aviv): Cinematography and Scanning Electron Microscopy of Leukocytic Rings Formed *in vitro* Around *Cryptococcus neoformans* 60
Male, O. (Vienna): Pathogenesis of Mucocutaneous Mycoses Caused by Yeasts 66
Abramovici, A. (Petah-Tiqva): Mycotoxins and Abnormal Fetal Development 81
Kaufman, L. (Atlanta, Ga.): Immunology: Its Value in Diagnosing Systemic Fungal Infections 95
Levine, H.B.; Scalarone, G.M., and Chaparas, S.D. (Rockville, Md.): Preparation of Fungal Antigens and Vaccines: Studies on *Coccidioides immitis* and *Histoplasma Capsulatum* 106
Hasenclever, H.F. and McAtee, F.J. (Hamilton, Mont.): Antigenic Relationships of *Candida albicans, Saccharomyces telluris,* and *Saccharomyces cerevisiae* 126
Pine, L. (Atlanta, Ga.): Histoplasma Antigens: Their Production, Purification and Uses 138

Author Index 169
Subject Index 170

Host-Parasite Relationships in Systemic Mycoses
Part II: Specific Diseases and Therapy

Proceedings of the 21st Annual OHOLO Biological Conference, Ma'alot, Israel 1976, published as Vol. 4 of 'Contributions to Microbiology and Immunology'.

Conference Organizing Committee	VII
Acknowledgments	VIII
List of Participants	IX
Preface	XIII

Mariat, F.; Destombes, P., and Segretain, G. (Paris): The Mycetomas: Clinical Features, Pathology, Etiology and Epidemiology ... 1

Schnell, J.D. (Wuppertal): The Epidemiology and Prophylaxis of Mycoses in Perinatology ... 40

Kuttin, E.S. and Beemer, A.M. (Ness-Ziona): Systemic Mycoses in Israel ... 46

Bulmer, C. (Jerusalem): The Ocular Mycoses ... 56

Winner, H.I. (London): Recent Advances in Systemic Candidosis ... 64

Iwata, K. (Tokyo): Toxins Produced by *Candida albicans* ... 77

Seeliger, H.P.R. (Würzburg): Cryptococcosis: A Diagnostic Challenge ... 86

Baum, G.L. (Tel-Aviv) and *Schwarz, J.* (Cincinnati, Ohio): Histoplasmosis ... 96

Einstein, H.E. (Los Angeles, Calif.): Coccidioidomycosis and Blastomycosis ... 108

Loeffler, W. (Basel): Antifungal Agents ... 113

Utz, J.P. (Washington, D.C.): The Current Status of Chemotherapeutic Agents for the Systemic Mycoses ... 124

Beemer, A.M.; Kuttin, E.S., and Pinto, M. (Ness-Ziona): Treatment with Antifungal Vaccines ... 136

Shadomy, S. (Richmond, Va.): *In vitro* and *In vivo* Studies on Synergistic Antifungal Activity ... 147

Polak, A. (Basel): 5-Fluorocytosine-Current Status with Special References to Mode of Action and Drug Resistance ... 158

Round Table Discussion	168
Author Index	186
Subject Index	187

Conference Organizing Committee

Dr. Eliezer S. Kuttin, Israel Institute for Biological Research, Ness-Ziona (Chairman of the Committee)
Dr. Chaim Almog, Asaf Harofeh Government Hospital, Zerifin, and Tel-Aviv University Sackler School of Medicine, Tel-Aviv
Dr. Avraham M. Beemer, Israel Institute for Biological Research, Ness-Ziona
Dr. Amnon Ben-David, Israel Institute for Biological Research, Ness-Ziona
Dr. Ruth Corett, Israel Institute for Biological Research, Ness-Ziona
Dr. Salomon Ganor, Jerusalem
Prof. Nathan Grossowicz, Hebrew University, Jerusalem
Prof. Alexander Keynan, Hebrew University, Jerusalem
Prof. Marcus A. Klingberg, Israel Institute for Biological Research, Ness-Ziona, and Tel-Aviv University Sackler School of Medicine, Tel-Aviv
Prof. Alexander Kohn, Israel Institute for Biological Research, Ness-Ziona and Tel-Aviv University Sackler School of Medicine, Tel-Aviv
Prof. Emmanuel Levy, The Hospital of the Emek Medical Center, Afula, and Aba Khoushy School of Medicine, The Technion, Haifa
Prof. Henry N. Neufeld, Chaim Sheba Medical Centre, Tel-Hashomer, and Tel-Aviv University Sackler School of Medicine, Tel-Aviv
Dr. Moshe Pinto, Israel Institute for Biological Research, Ness-Ziona
Prof. Michael Sela, Weizmann Institute of Science, Rehovot
Mrs. Myra Kaye, Scientific Secretary to the Committee, Ness-Ziona
Miss Haya Bart, Organizing Secretary, Ness-Ziona
Mr. Chanoh Yorav, Technical Organizer, Ness-Ziona

Acknowledgments

A Conference organized and sponsored by the *Israel Institute for Biological Research* Ness-Ziona, Israel
affiliated to the Tel-Aviv University Sackler School of Medicine

The financial support given to the conference by the following institutions is gratefully acknowledged:

Austrian Embassy, Tel-Aviv (Israel)
Bayer AG, Leverkusen (FRG)
The British Council
Carl-Zeiss Company, Oberkoehen (FRG)
Discount Bank, Ltd., Tel-Aviv (Israel)
El Al Israel Airlines
Fischer Pharmaceuticals Ltd., Tel-Aviv (Israel)
French Embassy, Tel-Aviv (Israel)
Bank Hapoalim Ltd., Tel-Aviv (Israel)
Israel Cancer Association, Tel-Aviv (Israel)
M.A.I. Ltd., Jerusalem (Israel)
Monaghan Division, Monaghan Company, (USA)
Patra Travel Agency Ltd., Tel-Aviv (Israel)
E.R. Squibb and Sons, Ltd. (England)
Dr. August Wolff, Chem. Pharm. Fabrik, K.G., Bielefeld (FRG)

List of Participants

Ajello, L., Center for Disease Control, Atlanta, Ga. (USA)
Akov, Y., Israel Institute for Biological Research, Ness-Ziona (Israel)
Akov, Shoshana, Israel Institute for Biological Research, Ness-Ziona (Israel)
Almog, C., Asaf Harofeh Government Hospital, Zerifin (Israel)
Altstock, W., Abic Ltd., Ramat Gan (Israel)
Ansehn, S., University of Linköping, Linköping (Sweden)
Avigad, J., Rockach Hospital (Hadassah) Tel-Aviv (Israel)
Austwick, P.K.C., Nuffield Institute of Comparative Medicine, London (England)
Bart, Haya, Israel Institute for Biological Research, Ness-Ziona (Israel)
Baum, G.L., Chaim Sheba Medical Center, Tel-Hashomer (Israel)
Beemer, A.M., Israel Institute for Biological Research, Ness-Ziona (Israel)
Ben-David, A., Israel Institute for Biological Research, Ness-Ziona (Israel)
Bergman, S., University of Linköping, Linköping (Sweden)
Berdicevsky, Israela, Aba Khoushy School of Medicine, Technion, Haifa (Israel)
Bitron, Aviva, Israel Institute for Biological Research, Ness-Ziona (Israel)
Bulmer, Caryl, Hadassah University Hospital, Jerusalem (Israel)
Corett, Ruth, Israel Institute for Biological Research, Ness-Ziona (Israel)
Duvedevani, Nurit, Israel Institute for Biological Research, Ness-Ziona (Israel)
Einstein, H.E., University of Southern California, School of Medicine, Los Angeles, Calif. (USA)
Elian, Inge, Hasharon Hospital, Petah-Tiqva (Israel)
Elian, M., National Worker's Sick Fund (Israel)
Evenchik, Z., Israel Institute for Biological Research, Ness-Ziona (Israel)
Folb, P., Chaim Sheba Medical Center, Tel-Hashomer (Israel)
Fuchs, P., Israel Institute for Biological Research, Ness-Ziona (Israel)
Ganor, S., 23, Keren Hayesod St., Jerusalem (Israel)
Gerichter, C., Government Central Laboratories, Ministry of Health, Jerusalem (Israel)
Goldstein, Dinah, Hebrew University-Hadassah Medical School, Jerusalem (Israel)
Goldwasser, R.A., Israel Institute for Biological Research, Ness-Ziona (Israel)
Grossowicz, N., Hebrew University-Hadassah Medical School, Jerusalem (Israel)
Hasenclever, H.F., National Institute of Allergy and Infectious Diseases, Hamilton, Mont. (USA)
Halmann, Mirjam, Israel Institute for Biological Research, Ness-Ziona (Israel)
Haimson, Michal, Israel Institute for Biological Research, Ness-Ziona (Israel)
Hecht, B., Israel Institute for Biological Research, Ness-Ziona (Israel)

List of Participants

Henig, E., Beilinson Hospital, Petah-Tiqva (Israel)
Herzog, Naomi, Hadassah University Hospital, Jerusalem (Israel)
Iwata, K., University of Tokyo, School of Medicine, Tokyo (Japan)
Kaplan, W., Center for Disease Control, Atlanta, Ga. (USA)
Katz, D., Israel Institute for Biological Research, Ness-Ziona (Israel)
Katzenelbogen, Orit, Israel Institute for Biological Research, Ness-Ziona (Israel)
Kaufman, L., Center for Disease Control, Atlanta, Ga. (USA)
Kaye, Myra, Israel Institute for Biological Research, Ness-Ziona (Israel)
Kejzman, G., Abic Ltd., Ramat-Gan (Israel)
Kletter, Yehudith, Tel-Aviv University, Sackler School of Medicine, Tel-Aviv (Israel)
Klibansky, T., Israel Institute for Biological Research, Ness-Ziona (Israel)
Klingberg, M.A., Israel Institute for Biological Research, Ness-Ziona (Israel)
Klingberg, Wanda, Israel Institute for Biological Research, Ness-Ziona (Israel)
Köhler, H., Tierärztliche Hochschule in Wien, Vienna (Austria)
Kohn, A., Israel Institute for Biological Research, Ness-Ziona (Israel)
Kohn, Hanna, Sick Fund of the General Labor Federation, Rehovot (Israel)
Kuttin, E.S., Israel Institute for Biological Research, Ness-Ziona (Israel)
Lehrer, Nurit, Beilinson Hospital, Petah Tiqva (Israel)
Levine, H.B., University of California, Naval Supply Center, Oakland, Ca. (USA)
Löbel, Esther, Weizmann Institute of Science, Rehovot (Israel)
Loeffler, W., University of Tübingen, Tübingen (FRG)
Louria, D.B., New Jersey Medical School, Newark, N.J. (USA)
Lutzky, I., Hebrew University-Hadassah Medical School, Jerusalem (Israel)
Male, O., Allgemeines Krankenhaus der Stadt Wien, Vienna (Austria)
Margalit, Y., Israel Institute for Biological Research, Ness-Ziona (Israel)
Mariat, F., Institut Pasteur, Paris (France)
Mates, H., Poria Government Hospital, Tiberias (Israel)
Mendes, M., Center for Prevention of Lung Diseases, Tel-Aviv (Israel)
Merzbach, D., Rambam Hospital and Aba Khoushy Medical School, Haifa (Israel)
Meshulam, M., Israel Institute for Biological Research, Ness-Ziona (Israel)
Mielnick, Maria, Coney Island Hospital, New York, N.Y. (USA)
Paretsky, D., Hebrew University-Hadassah Medical School, Jerusalem (Israel)
Peleg, J., Israel Institute for Biological Research, Ness-Ziona (Israel)
Pine, L., Center for Disease Control, Atlanta, Ga.(USA)
Pinto, M., Israel Institute for Biological Research, Ness-Ziona (Israel)
Plempel, M., Institut fur Chemotherapie, Bayer Forschungszentrum, Wuppertal (FRG)
Polacheck, I., Hebrew University, Jerusalem (Israel)
Polak, Annemarie, F. Hoffmann-La Roche and Co., A.G., Basel (Switzerland)
Rabinowitz, Sonya, Government Central Laboratories, Ministry of Health, Jerusalem (Israel)
Rachmuth, Pepi, Beilinson Hospital, Petah-Tiqva (Israel)
Raubitschek, Hella, Hadassah University Hospital, Jerusalem (Israel)
Sacks, T., Hebrew University-Hadassah Medical School and Hadassah University Hospital, Jerusalem (Israel)
Schnell, J., Rheinische Land Klinik, Wuppertal (FRG)
Seeliger, H., Universitat Würzburg, Würzburg (FRG)
Seligmann, Rachel, Public Health Laboratory, Ministry of Health, Haifa (Israel)
Shahar, A., Israel Institute for Biological Research, Ness-Ziona (Israel)
Shapiro-Hirsch, Raya, Sick Fund of the General Labor Federation, Haifa (Israel)
Simon, G., Israel Institute for Biological Research, Ness-Ziona (Israel)
Simonovitch, C., Abic Ltd., Ramat-Gan Israel

List of Participants

Sommer, B., Chaim Sheba Medical Center, Tel-Hashomer (Israel)
Sporn, Jaffa, Beilinson Hospital, Petah-Tiqva (Israel)
Staib, F., Robert Koch-Institut des Bundesgesundheitsamtes, Berlin (FRG)
Stein, Bela., Sick Fund of the General Labor Federation, Tel-Aviv (Israel)
Steinbock, D., Israel Institute for Biological Research, Ness-Ziona (Israel)
Stettendorf, Siegfried, Bayer, A.G., Leverkusen (FRG)
Straussman, Yoheved, Israel Institute for Biological Research, Ness-Ziona (Israel)
Tonolo, A., Istituto Superiore di Sanita, Roma (Italy)
Tortorano, Anna-Maria, Istituto D'Igiene della Universita' Di Milano, Milano (Italy)
Uchovsky, D., Hadera (Israel)
Ungar, H., Hebrew University-Hadassah Medical School, and Hadassah Hospital, Jerusalem (Israel)
Utz, J.P., Georgetown University School of Medicine, Washington, D.C. (USA)
Viviani, Maria-Anna, Istituto D'Igiene della Universita' Di Milano, Milano (Italy)
Wegmann, T., Klinik A für Innere Medizin, Kantonsspital, St. Gallen (Switzerland)
Weidenfeld, Lily, Tel-Aviv (Israel)
Yathom, Shulamith, Sick Fund of the General Labor Federation, Tel-Aviv (Israel)
Yorav, C., Israel Institute for Biological Research, Ness-Ziona (Israel)
Zaltser, Hayuta, Sick Fund of the General Labor Federation, Haifa (Israel)
Feldmann, Z., Health District Office, Ministry of Health, Petah-Tiqva (Israel)
Feldmann, Miriam, Medical Corps, Israel Defence Forces
Richards, M., Beecham Pharmaceuticals, Surrey (England)
Shadomy, S., Medical College of Virginia, Richmond, Va. (USA)
Shalish, Lea, Chaim Sheba Medical Center, Tel-Hashomer (Israel)

Preface

The OHOLO Conferences have been convened annually since the Spring of 1956. They have covered very wide areas from different and overlapping disciplines.

The participants at these meetings, from many countries as well as from different scientific institutions in Israel, are engaged in fields of study which represent widely divergent approaches to biology. Thus, a characteristic feature of the OHOLO meetings has been their multi-disciplinary nature.

These small international conferences are distinguished by the relaxed atmosphere in which they are held, with ample time for informal as well as formal discussions.

The 21st OHOLO Biological Conference, on "Host Parasite Relationships in Systemic Mycoses", opened the third decade of OHOLO Conferences. In the many topics covered in the twenty previous conferences, and in spite of changes in location, membership of the organising committees and the attending participants, the main idea of the "founding fathers" of the OHOLO conferences remains unchanged: to bring together Israeli and foreign scientists and students, in order to promote and encourage interdisciplinary research in fields that are in the forefront of scientific advance and interest.

When Host-Parasite Relationships in Systemic Mycoses was proposed to the permanent OHOLO committee as the topic for the 1976 OHOLO conference, it was unanimously and enthusiastically accepted. The systemic, or deep mycoses, hold today a special place in the large spectrum of infectious diseases. Medical progress, in particular the introduction of chemotherapy and vaccination, has changed drastically the role of infectious diseases as a major cause of morbidity and mortality in developed countries. However, as far as the mycoses are concerned, medical progress has been associated with an increase in their incidence and severity. In spite of this, regrettably, basic and applied research devoted to medically important fungi and the diseases they cause are not as fashionable as is research in other areas in medicine and microbiology. The scarcity of antimycotic agents for treatment is perhaps not only a result of the peculiarities of fungi, but also a reflection of the insufficient efforts invested in research in this field, as compared to the huge efforts applied to curb other infectious diseases.

The aim of the Conference was to bring together scientists and clinicians, and to find the right balance between the presentation of clinical information and of research findings on basic biological mechanisms related to the host-parasite relationship. It was our intention to widen rather than to limit the scope of the discussions: Thus some papers were included which might not strictly be in place under the subject title of the Conference; however, it was our feeling that they would represent the wider outlook which is essential for the understanding of biological systems.

Although the problems of host-parasite relationships in the systemic mycoses were discussed, referred to or form the background of all the papers, it was in the Round Table Discussion, traditionally held at the end of OHOLO meetings and chaired on this occasion by Professor *Utz*, that the paramount issues relating to this topic were dealt with both specifically and widely. We have endeavored to present the discussion as faithfully as possible in spirit and content. Although a number of questions raised in the conference were answered, more importantly, new questions and ideas to inspire future work emerged as a result of our OHOLO meetings.

The papers published here are divided into two volumes, and arranged under the subtitles "Methodology, pathology and immunology" (part I), and "Specific diseases and therapy" (including also the Round Table Discussion) (part II). This arrangement is somewhat arbitrary, since many participants discussed various aspects which would fall into either category. Some overlap is therefore inevitable.

The Editors gladly take this opportunity to express their thanks to the Organizing Committee and its Officers for their efforts and dedication in preparing the meeting. We also express our gratitude to the supplementary staff, Ms. *Nurit Duvdevani* and *Orit Katzenelenbogen* for also giving freely of their time in the preparatory work and for their invaluable secretarial services during the Conference.

We thank also the management and staff of the Ma'alot Guest House for their care of our guests.

The Editors

Introductory Remarks

It was twenty years ago that the first Biological Conference organized and sponsored by the Israel Institute for Biological Research took place in an educational center called "OHOLO", on the shores of Lake Kinnereth. Hence the name, in case some of you wondered about it. The name OHOLO is connected with the history of the Labour Movement in Israel, but the twenty conferences held since 1956 gave the name OHOLO an extra meaning, and even though the Conferences are no longer held in the original OHOLO center, they are still and will remain the OHOLO Biological Conferences.

The topic of the 1976 meeting was unanimously adopted by the Permanent OHOLO Committee. I do not have to convince this audience of the importance of fungi. The fact that fungi are now classified as a kingdom signifies the special characteristics of these organisms and also our growing awareness of their importance in various fields.

The topic of this meeting is basically an ecological problem – the interaction between the fungi and animal kingdoms, and in particular the situation where there is a disturbance in equilibrium, resulting in a systemic mycosis. As in other ecological systems, progress and solutions to certain problems lead to the emergence of new ones. The progress made in the fields of antibiotic therapy, the treatment of cancer, and organ transplantation, also brought systemic mycoses into the limelight, with all the grave problems of diagnosis and treatment that they pose.

Although I am sure that our honoured guests, who are among the most distinguished investigators in the field, and have had numerous other opportunities to meet, will also gain from this Conference, it is mainly we who are to profit. It is our hope that this Conference will promote understanding of the problems involved, and will stimulate future work in all the disciplines represented here.

I wish us all a pleasant and productive meeting and I invite Dr. Ajello to give the opening lecture of the Conference, on "Systematic Mycoses in Modern Medicine".

A. Ben-David
Israel Institute for Biological Research, Ness-Ziona

Systemic Mycoses in Modern Medicine

L. Ajello

Mycology Division, Center for Disease Control, Public Health Service, U.S. Department of Health, Education, and Welfare, Atlanta, Ga.

Despite the long history of medical mycology, one that covers a span of some 140 years, unlike many bacterial and viral diseases, no mycotic disease has been conquered.

Systemic infections caused by fungi constitute a major public health problem in many parts of the world, both in developed as well as third world countries. Paradoxically, some of the mycoses are most prevalent and have a higher incidence in the most medically advanced nations. We may very well ask then, why do we still have to contend with the variety of mycotic diseases that afflict literally millions of people and bring about the untimely death of unknown numbers of our fellow men?

The reasons for their persistence, and, in some instances for an increase in their prevalence, are quite diverse. Some have a historical basis, while others stem from the most dramatic achievements of modern medicine or from the very nature of the pathogenic fungi themselves.

Historically, the discovery of the etiologic role played by fungi in disease marked the very beginning of medical microbiology. The founder of the doctrine of pathogenic microbes was *Agostino Bassi*, a precursor of *Pasteur* and *Koch* (*Bulloch*, 1938). In 1835 *Bassi* revealed for the first time ever that a microorganism caused a disease. The etiologic agent was a mould, now known as *Beauvaria bassiana*. Publication of his epochal treatise, "Del Mal del Segno," on the cause and prevention of a devastating silk worm disease, was quickly followed by the first discoveries of human diseases caused by microbes, all fungi, eg. favus by *Remak* and *Schoenlein* in 1837 and 1842, respectively (*Kisch*, 1954), candidosis by *Gruby* in 1842, and aspergillosis by *Sluyter* in 1847. These fundamental discoveries antedated the era of medical bacteriology ushered in by the monumental work of *Pasteur* and his contemporaries in the 1860's.

Despite the prior discovery of mycotic diseases, their study was all but forgotten with the stark realization that the most prevalent and devastating diseases of man — plague, pneumonia, syphilis and tuberculosis, to name but a few — were caused by bacteria. These, and many other bacterial as well as parasitic and viral diseases were the major killers of the young and the old, the strong and the feeble, the rich and the poor. Until the other microbial diseases were conquered or controlled by improvements in sanitation, personal hygiene, nutrition, therapy and vaccines, the mycoses received little, if any, attention.

Aside from the pressing demands of the non-mycotic diseases, the fact that the science of medical mycology had a European origin, I believe, also served to hold down interest in the mycoses. As nature would have it, the European continent is completely free of the pathogenic fungi *Blastomyces dermatitidis, Coccidioides immitis* and *Paracoccidioides brasiliensis.* When present, the systemic pathogenic fungi are found in restricted areas and do not affect many individuals, as for example *Histoplasma capsulatum (Ajello,* 1967). Elsewhere, all of these fungi are important causes of morbidity and mortality. Had these fungi flourished in Europe, as they do in the Americas, Africa or Asia, the fungi may not have been so readily disregarded as disease agents and virtually forgotten.

This neglect of the systemic mycoses has persisted into our own era, aided and abetted by lapses in the education and training of medical and paramedical professionals. In too many medical institutions and universities, medical mycology is either not taught at all, or is treated in only a cursory manner. This dearth of training inevitably leads to misdiagnosis and mistreatment of mycotic diseases, with dire consequences to patients. The fact that the systemic mycoses mimic other diseases in their clinical and pathological expression is worsened by diagnostic ignorance. With adequate training in the clinical signs of the mycoses, in the methodology needed to diagnose them and in their therapy, the public health burden imposed on mankind by the pathogenic fungi could be materially reduced.

This has happened in the United States, where dissemination of knowledge concerning the diagnosis and treatment of blastomycosis has almost ended fatalities due to *B. dermatitides;* over the decade 1964—1973,[1] the annual deaths due to this fungus ranged from a high of 29 to a low of none. In 1968, 1972 and 1973 no blastomycosis deaths were recorded, and in 1969, 1970 and 1971, deaths due to this disease were only 2, 3 and 3 respectively. Mortality due to *C. immitis* and *H. capsulatum* also showed a tendency to decrease during that decade, but to a much lesser extent.

In contrast, deaths ascribed to candidosis and cryptococcosis have increased rather than diminished. Here, the heightened mortality is in all probability a reflection of the opportunism of *Candida albicans* and *Cryptococcus neoformans,* coupled with modern methods of treating infections and other diseases.

[1] Latest year with available data (Morbidity and Mortality, 1975).

For, as contradictory as it may at first seem, the introduction and widespread use of therapeutic agents such as antibiotics, corticosteroids, immunosuppressants and radiation have made the recipients of these therapeutic measures vulnerable to superimposed mycotic infections. Not only are *C. albicans* and *C. neoformans* involved, but also a seemingly unending series of fungi previously not known to be pathogenic to man (*Drouhet*, 1970).

The increase in man's longevity has resulted in an increase in the prevalence and incidence of chronic degenerative and neoplastic diseases. Individuals with these diseases frequently have insult added to injury by the development of secondary and often lethal mycotic infections, such as aspergillosis, candidosis, cryptococcosis, phaeohyphomycosis (*Ajello*, 1975) and zygomycosis.

Tragically, just how many patients are victims of opportunistic fungi, or, for that matter, how many cases of systemic fungus disease occur in any country is not known. Not a single country in the entire world has realized the necessity of making mycotic diseases notifiable to a public health agency. As a result of this lapse in responsibility, public health workers lack vital statistics on the incidence and prevalence of mycotic diseases or on the mortality that they cause.[2] Without such data, support for medical mycological teaching, training and diagnostic centers, as well as basic and applied research is difficult to justify and funding difficult to obtain from administrators. Medical mycologists must compete for support from a limited pool of funds against investigators of all other diseases. But the others, being notifiable, are backed up by data on morbidity and mortality that sway the minds of men and loosen purse strings.

It is frustrating for those who work in medical mycology to know that the mycoses are not rare and that control programs cry for support. A rare and revealing insight into the incidence and public health impact of the systemic mycoses within the United States was provided recently by a computerized analysis of hospital records. This study by *Hammerman et al.* (1974) revealed the following data for the year 1970: Patients hospitalized with diagnoses of blastomycosis, candidosis, coccidioidomycosis, cryptococcosis or histoplasmosis totaled 6,868. Deaths due to these five diseases were, through extrapolation, determined to total 263. This proved to be an underestimation of reality. For 1970, the Center for Disease Control reported that 365 deaths had been attributed to these five mycoses (Morbidity and Mortality, 1975).

Other computations and extrapolations of the base data provided estimates of 500,000 annual infections by *H. capsulatum*, 200,000 of those victims becoming clinically ill and 4,000 requiring hospitalization. The figures for coccidioidomycosis were 100,000 infections, 40,000 clinically ill and 2,000 hospital-

---

[2] The mortality figures quoted previously on blastomycosis in the United States came from a listing of deaths from selected non-notifiable diseases compiled originally from death certificates.

izations. Reported deaths due to these diseases for 1970 were 56 for histoplasmosis and 42 for coccidioidomycosis.

The persistence of the systemic mycoses involves also ecological factors. Among the six most prevalent mycoses, five are known or are presumed to be caused by fungi that live and flourish as saprophytes in the environment. Although the specific habitats of *B. dermatitidis* and *P. brasiliensis* have not been discovered, all clinical and epidemiological evidence points to a saprophytic existence in nature. Their ecological requirements must be quite special since all attempts to uncover and define them, so far, have ended in failure.

The natural habitats of *C. immitis, C. neoformans* and *H. capsulatum* are more or less defined. *C. immitis* is a geophilic mould confined to the New World and adapted to live specifically in the desert-like terrain of North, Central and South America (*Ajello,* 1967). The separation of the American continents from Europe, Africa, and Asia by the geologic movement of tectonic plates may be presumed to have played a crucial role in confining this pathogenic fungus to the New World.

C. neoformans is a cosmopolitan basidomycetous yeast (*Kwon-Chung,* 1975) that multiplies extraordinarily well in the feces-enriched nests of pigeons (*Columba liva*). A high percentage of the nests of the bird, in both rural and urban sites, harbor as many as 50,000,000 cells/g of *C. neoformans* (*Emmons,* 1962).

H. capsulatum also has a worldwide distribution. But, here again, the fungus does not occur at random in soil. It is most commonly found and flourishes most abundantly in bat and bird habitats.

In contrast to these five geophilic fungi, *C. albicans* exists as a commensal in the bodies of humans and other animals. Normally a balance exists between the host and its potential parasite, but when this equilibrium is broken by internal or external factors, the yeast multiplies wildly and its millions of cells invade and destroy vital tissue.

Infectious fungus cells thus abound in and around us, and it is not foreseeable at this time how their potential threat can be eliminated or reduced. Practical and economical means to sterilize the natural habitats of the geophilic fungi have not been developed and the magnitude of the problem boggles the mind. The threat posed by commensal fungi also has not been met. In modern medicine, the systemic mycoses remain a challenge and an inspiration to greater effort to understand them and to minimize the toll that they extract from us in terms of misery, death and economic loss.

Toward this end we must all join in a concerted drive to make the mycoses notifiable. Once the magnitude of the problem that we all sense is backed by hard facts and figures, the mycoses will gain the long overdue attention of the public, government and research administrators, as well as educators and scientists. If there will be a sustained effort in this direction, we can all look forward to the day when diagnostic acumen is widespread, physicians have at their disposal a battery of specific and effective therapeutic agents to administer, and vaccines, as well as other preventive measures, have been perfected and put to use.

International meetings in different parts of the world, such as this OHOLO Conference, not only serve to update the knowledge of the participants already interested in medical mycology, but they also serve to publicize developments and problems and educate others to realize the importance of the mycoses in public health.

References

Ajello, L.: Comparative ecology of respiratory mycotic disease agents. Bact. Rev. *31:* 6–24 (1967).
Ajello, L.: Phaeohyphomycosis: definition and etiology. Proc. 3rd Int. Conf. Mycoses. Sci. Publ. No. 304 (Pan American Health Organization, Washington 1975).
Bassi, A.: Del Mal del Segno; in *Ainsworth* Phytopathological Classic No. 10 (Am. Phytopath. Soc., Baltimore 1958).
Bulloch, W.: The history of bacteriology (Oxford University Press, London 1938).
Drouhet, E.: Champignons opportunistes et mycoses iatrogènes. Bull. Inst. Pasteur *70:* 391–464 (1970).
Emmons, C.W.: Natural occurrence of opportunistic fungi. J. Lab. Invest. *11:* 1026–1032 (1962).
Gruby, D.: Recherches anatomiques sur une plante cryptograme qui constitue le vraie muguet des enfants. C. hebd. Séanc. Acad. Sci., Paris *14:* 634–636 (1842).
Hammerman, K.J.; Powell, K.E., and Tosh, F.E.: The incidence of hospitalized cases of systemic mycotic infection. Sabouraudia *12:* 33–45 (1974).
Kisch, B.: Forgotten leaders in modern medicine: Valentin, Gruby, Remak, Auerbach. Trans. Am. Philos. Soc. *44/2:* 139–317 (1954).
Kwon-Chung, K.J.: A new genus, *Filobasidiella,* the perfect state of *Cryptococcus neoformans.* Mycologia *67:* 1197–1200 (1975).
Morbidity and Mortality. Weekly report for year ending Dec. 28, 1974, vol. 23, pp. 1–60 (Center for Disease Control, Public Health Service, Atlanta 1975).
Sluyter, T.: De vegetabilibus organismi animalis parasitis ac de novo epiphyto in pityriasi versicolor obvio; thesis Berlin (1847).

Dr. *L. Ajello,* Mycology Division, Center for Disease Control, Public Health Service, U.S. Department of Health, Education and Welfare, *Atlanta, GA 30333* (USA)

Medically Important Infectious Fungi

L. Ajello

Mycology Division, Center for Disease Control, Public Health Service, U.S. Department of Health, Education, and Welfare, Atlanta, Ga.

Introduction

Broad topics such as the one that we have before us can be dealt with in diverse ways. In a clinical approach, the pathogenic fungi could be grouped and discussed on the basis of the type of disease that they induce in their hosts: superficial, cutaneous, subcutaneous or systemic. Another possible approach, and the one that I have selected, would be basically taxonomic, rather than clinical, in its exposition. My choice was governed by the feeling that many clinicians and even some mycologists have not kept up with the radical changes that have taken place in the classic treatment of the fungi as members of the Plant Kingdom (table I) and of the Division Thallophyta (table II). The fungi have not only been separated from the algae, with which they were linked in the

Table I. Classical treatment of the plant kingdom

Divisions	Components
Spermatophyta	seed plants
Pteridophyta	ferns and fern allies
Bryophyta	mosses and liverworts
Thallophyta	algae and fungi

Table II. Classification of the obsolete division Thallophyta

Algae	Fungi
Chlorophyceae	Basidiomycetes
Rhodophyceae	Ascomycetes
	Phycomycetes
	Schizomycetes

Thallophyta, but they have been withdrawn from the Plant Kingdom and placed in one of their very own. Contemporary taxonomists no longer consider the fungi to be plants. Phylogenetically, they are considered to be so distinct and divergent that the Kingdom, Fungi, has been created to accommodate them (*Whittaker*, 1969).

For the purposes of this publication, we have chosen to follow *Ainsworth's* (1971, 1973) classification scheme in dealing with the fungi that cause human disease. In his concept, the organisms considered to be fungi are dealt with as follows.

Kingdom: Fungi

Division I: Myxomycota

All fungi with their basic structure in the form of a plasmodium or pseudoplasmodium.
Classes
  1. Acrasiomycetes
Free-living myxamoebae that aggregate to form a pseudoplasmodium prior to reproduction
  2. Labyrinthulales
Fungi whose basic structure is a net-like plasmodium
  3. Myxomycetes
Fungi whose basic structure is a free-living plasmodium that does not form a network
  4. Plasmodiophoromycetes
Fungi whose basic structure is a parasitic plasmodium found within the cells of plants.

Division II: Eumycota

The true fungi. Plasmodia or pseudoplasmodia not formed. Assimilative phase, filamentous (with some important exceptions).

Subdivisions
A. Mastigomycotina
Zoospores produced. Oospores produced in perfect state
Classes
  1. Chytridiomycetes
Zoospores with a single posterior whiplash-type flagellum
  2. Hyphochytridiomycetes
Zoospores with a single anterior tinsel-type flagellum

3. Oomycetes
Biflagellate zoospores: Anterior tinsel-type flagellum; posterior whiplash-type flagellum

B. Zygomycotina
Motile spores not produced, mycelium, when present, aseptate.
Perfect state characterized by production of zygospores
Classes

1. Zygomycetes
Saprophytic, parasitic or predaceous. Mycelium immersed in host tissue when parasitic or predaceous

2. Trichomycetes
Found associated with arthropods; attached to their cuticle or gut by a holdfast. Not immersed in host tissue

C. Ascomycotina
Ascospores characteristic of perfect state. Mycelium, if present, septate
Classes

1. Hemiascomycetes
Ascocarps and ascogenous hyphae not produced. Mycelial and unicellular forms.

2. Loculoascomycetes
Ascocarps and ascogenous hyphae produced. Asci bitunicate, ascocarp an ascostroma

3. Plectomycetes
Ascocarps and ascogenous hyphae produced. Asci typically unitunicate; if bitunicate, ascocarp is an apothecium. Asci evanescest, scattered within cleistothecia. Ascospores unicellular

4. Laboulbeniomycetes
Asci regularly arranged within the ascocarp in a basal or peripheral layer. Exoparasites of arthropods

5. Pyrenomycetes
Ascocarp a perithecium usually with an ostiole, asci inoperculate, ascocpores discharged through an apical pore or slit.

6. Discomycetes
Ascocarps apothecia on ground or underground. Asci with or without operculi.

D. Basidiomycotina
Basidiospores characteristic of perfect state. Mycelium, if present, septate.
Classes

1. Teliomycetes

Basidiocarps not produced. Teliospores usually in host tissue. Most species parasitic in vascular plants

    2. Hymenomycetes

Fungi that form basidiocarps. Basidia forming a hymenium. Saprophytic or parasitic. Basidiocarps gymnocarpous or semiangiocarpous. Basidia septate or aseptate. Basidiospores ballistospores

    3. Gasteromycetes

Fungi with angiocarpous basidiocarps. Basidia aseptate; basidiospores not ballistospores

E. Deuteromycotina

Filamentous or unicellular fungi without a perfect state or, if present, generally encountered in their imperfect state

Classes

    1. Blastomycetes

Basically unicellular fungi that reproduce by a budding process. Mycelium or pseudomycelium may or may not be produced

    2. Hyphomycetes

Septate mycelium produced that may be sterile or bears conidia on conidiophores that are not within acervuli or pycnidia

    3. Coelomycetes

Mycelium septate – conidia borne in acervuli or pycnidia.

The fungi currently known to infect man and other mammals and birds are all members of the Division Eumycota. Pathogenic species are found in the subdivisions Zygomycotina, Ascomycotina, Basidiomycotina and Deuteromycotina. As yet none have been found in the subdivision Mastigomycotina. It should be noted however that recently *Austwick and Copland* (1974) suggested that *Hyphomyces destruens,* the agent of an equine disease referred to as "swamp cancer," is not a zygomycete but rather a species of *Pythium.* If that report is confirmed, the subdivision Mastigomycotina will enter the province of medical mycology. The genus *Pythium* is classified in that subdivision in the class Oomycetes, in the order Peronosporales, and in the family Pythiaceae.

Tables III–VIII list the most common of the pathogenic fungi by Subdivision, Class, Order, Family, Genus and Species. In table III it will be noted that three pathogenic zygomycetes classified in two genera are members of the order Entomophthorales. In contrast, the order Mucorales has 6 genera and 10 species of pathogenic fungi (*Ajello et al.,* 1975; *Carter et al.,* 1973).

The Subdivision Ascomycotina contains almost all of the pathogenic fungi that have been discovered to have a perfect or sexual state (table IV).

Among the basidiomycetes, only three species are documented sufficiently well to be considered pathogenic to man. These are *Coprinus cinereus (Speller*

Table III. Genera and pathogenic species of the subdivision Zygomycotina

Class: Zygomycetes
  Order: Entomophthorales
    Family: Entomophthoraceae
      Genus: Basidiobolus
        Species: B. haptosporus
      Genus: Conidiobolus
        Species: C. coronata
                 C. incongruus
  Order: Mucorales
    Family: Mucoraceae
      Genus: Abisida
        Species: A. corymbifera
      Genus: Cunninghamella
        Species: C. elegans

Genus: Mortierella
  Species: M. wolfii
Genus: Mucor
  Species: M. pusillus
           M. ramosissimus
Genus: Rhizopus
  Species: R. arrhizus
           R. microsporus
           R. oryzae
           R. rhizopodiformis
Family: Saksenaceae
  Genus: Saksenaea
    Species: S. vasiformis

Table IV. Genera and pathogenic species of the subdivision Ascomycotina

Class I. Hemiascomycetes
  Order: Endomycetales
    Family: Endomycetaceae
      Genus: Endomyces
        Species: E. candidus
                 (Geotichum candidum)[1]
                 (Butler and Petersen 1972)

    Family: Saccharomycetaceae
      Genus: Kluyveromyces
        Species: K. fragiles
                 (Candida pseudotropicalis)
      Genus: Pichia
        Species: P. guilliermondii
                 (C. guilliermondii)
        Species: P. kudriavzevii
                 (C. krusei)
      Genus: Loderomyces
        Species: L. elongosporus
                 (C. parapsilosis)

Class II. Loculoascomycetes
  Order: Myriangiales
    Family: Saccardinulaceae
      Genus: Piedraia
        Species: P. hortae
                 (Borelli 1959)

Order: Pleosporales
  Family: Pleosporaceae
    Genus: Cochliobolus
      Species: C. spicifer
  Family: Testudinaceae
    Genus: Neotestudina
      Species: N. rosatii
  Family: Zopfiaceae
    Genus: Zopfia
      Species: Z. senegalensis
               (Hawksworth and Booth 1974)
               Z. tompkinsii
  Family: Microascaceae
    Genus: Petriellidium
      Species: P. boydii
               (Malloch 1970)

Class III. Plectomycetes
  Order: Eurotiales
    Family: Gymnoascaceae
      Genus: Ajellomyces
        Species: A. dermatitidis
                 (Blastomyces dermatitidis)
                 (McDonough and Lewis 1968)
      Genus: Arthroderma
        Species: A. benhamiae
                 (Trichophyton mentagrophytes)

Table IV (continued)

Species: A. ciferii 　　(T. georgiae) 　A. flavescens 　　(T. flavescens) 　A. gertlerii 　　(T. vanbreuseghemii) 　A. gloriae 　　(T. gloriae) 　A. insingulare 　　(T. terrestre) 　A. lenticularum 　　(T. terrestre) 　A. quadrifidum 　　(T. terrestre) 　A. simii 　　(T. simii) 　A. uncinatum 　　(T. ajelloi) 　A. vanbreuseghemii 　　(T. mentagrophytes) Genus: Nannizzia 　Species: N. borellii 　　(Microsporum amazonicum) 　N. cajetanii 　　(M. cookei)	Species: N. fulva 　　(M. fulvum) 　N. grubyia 　　(M. vanbreuseghemii) 　N. gypsea 　　(M. gypseum) 　N. incurvata 　　(M. gypseum) 　N. obtusa 　　(M. nanum) 　N. otae (Hasegawa and Usui 1976) 　　(M. canis) 　N. persicolor 　　(M. persicolor) 　N. racemosa 　　(M. racemosum) Genus: Emmonsiella 　Species: E. capsulata 　　(Kwon-Chung 1972) 　　(Histoplasma capsulatum)

[1] Imperfect states in parentheses.

Table V. Genera and pathogenic species of the subdivision Basidiomycotina

Class: Teliomycetes 　Order: Ustilaginales 　　Family: Filobasidiaceae 　　　Genus: Filobasidiella 　　　　Species: F. neoformans 　　　　(Kwon-Chung 1975b) 　　　　(Cryptococcus neoformans)[1]	Class: Hymenomycetes 　Subclass: Holobasidiomycetidae 　　Order: Aphyllophorales 　　　Family: Schizophyllaceae 　　　　Genus: Schizophyllum 　　　　　Species: S. commune 　　Order: Agaricales 　　　Family: Coprinaceae 　　　　Genus: Coprinus 　　　　　Species: C. cinereus

[1] Imperfect state

Table VI. Genera and pathogenic species of the class Blastomycetes of the subdivision Deuteromycotina

Class: Blastomycetes
  Family: Cryptococcaceae
    Order[1]
      Genus: Candida
        Species: *C. albicans*
                C. guilliermondii
                C. krusei
                C. pseudotropicalis
                C. tropicalis
	Genus: Cryptococcus
	  Species: *C. neoformans*
	Genus: Pityrosporum
	  Species: *P. furfur*
	         P. pachydermatis
	Genus: Torulopsis
	  Species: *T. glabrata*
	Genus: Trichosporon
	  Species: *T. cutaneum*

[1] *Lodder* (1970) considered the imperfect yeasts to be too heterogenous to classify them in taxa other than genera and species. *Kreger-Van Rij* (1973) placed them in families.

and Maciver, 1971), *Filobasidiella neoformans* (*Kwon-Chung*, 1975b), and *Schizophyllum commune* (*Kligman*, 1950; *Restrepo et al.*, 1973). *Ustilago maydis* has been reported as a disease agent of humans (*Moore et al.*, 1946; *Preininger*, 1937), but the supporting data are unconvincing. The classification of the three pathogenic species is presented in table V.

The vast majority of the fungi known to cause infections in man and lower animals are members of the Subdivision Deuteromycotina. These fungi either are not known to have a perfect state or are generally encountered in an asexual mode of reproduction. When their perfect state is found, most prove to be ascomycetes, or, only rarely, basidiomycetes.

The Deuteromycotina have undergone a radical change in their classification. Traditionally they had been placed in the class Deuteromycetes and subdivided into five orders:

Order 1. Sphaeropsidales: Conidia borne in pycnidia.

Order 2. Melanconiales: Conidia borne in acervuli.

Order 3. Moniliales: Conidia borne free on conidiophores.

Order 4. Pseudosaccharomycetales: Yeast-like fungi, with or without pseudomycelium or true mycelium, that form blastospores.

Order 5. Mycelia Sterila: No reproductive spores formed.

Further subdivision of the Order Moniliales, where most of the pathogenic fungi were classified, led to the creation of four families to accommodate them.

1. Moniliaceae: Mycelium, conidiophores and conidia hyaline or bright colored.

2. Dematiaceae: Hyphae, conidiophores or conidia dark colored.

3. Stilbaceae: Fruiting hyphae united to form a coremium.

4. Tuberculariaceae: Fruiting hyphae united to form a sporodochium.

Table VII. Common genera and pathogenic species of the class Hyphomycetes of the subdivision Deuteromycotina

Genus: Acremonium
  Species: *A. falciforme*
    (*Gams* 1971)
    A. kiliense
    (*Gams* 1971)
    A. recifei
    (*Gams* 1971)
Genus: Acrotheca
  Species: *A. aquaspersa*
    (*Borelli* 1972)
Genus: Aspergillus
  Species: *A. flavus* group
    A. fumigatus group
    A. nidulans group
Genus: Blastomyces
  Species: *B. dermatitidis*
Genus: Chrysosporium
  Species: *C. parvum*
    (*Carmichael* 1962)
    C. parvum var. *crescens*
    (*Carmichael* 1962)
Genus: Cladosporium
  Species: *C. carrionii*
    C. trichoides
Genus: Coccidioides
  Species: *C. immitis*
Genus: Curvularia
  Species: *C. geniculata*
    C. lunata
    C. senegalensis
Genus: Dactylaria
  Species: *D. gallopava*
Genus: Drechslera
  Species: *D. hawaiiensis*
    D. spiciciferum
Genus: Exophiala
  Species: *E. salmonis*
    E. werneckii
    (*Arx* 1971)
Genus: Epidermophyton
  Species: *E. floccosum*
Genus: Fonsecaea
  Species: *F. compactum*
    F. pedrosoi
Genus: Fusarium
  Species: *F. oxysporum*
    F. solani
Genus: Geotrichum
  Species: *G. candidum*
Genus: Histoplasma
  Species: *H. capsulatum* var. *capsulatum*
    (*Kwon-Chung* 1972)
    H. capsulatum var. *duboisii*
    (*Kwon-Chung* 1975a)
    H. faiciminosum
Genus: Loboa
  Species: *L. loboi*
Genus: Madurella
  Species: *M. grisea*
    M. mycetomii
Genus: Microsporum
  Species: *M. amazonicum*
    M. audouinii
    M. boullardii
    M. canis
    M. cookei
    M. distortum
    M. equinum
    M. ferrugineum
    M. fulvum
    M. gypseum
    M. nanum
    M. persicolor
    M. praecox
    M. racemosum
    M. ripariae
    M. vanbreuseghemii
Genus: Paracoccidioides
  Species: *P. brasilienses*
Genus: Penicillium
  Species: *P. marneffei*
Genus: Phialophora
  Species: *P. gougerotii*
    P. jeanselmei
    P. mutabilis
    P. parasitica
    P. richardsiae
    P. spicifera
    P. verrucosa

Table VII (continued)

Genus: Prototheca	Genus: Trichophyton
Species: *P. wickerhamii*	Species: *T. longifusus*
P. zopfii	*T. megninii*
Genus: Rhinosporidium	*T. mentagrophytes* complex
Species: *R. seeberi*	*T.m.* var. *erinacei*
Genus: Sporothrix	*T.m.* var. *interdigitale*
Species: *schenckii*	*T.m.* var. *mentagrophytes*
Genus: Torula	*T.m.* var. *nodulare*
Species: *T. dermatitidis*	*T.m.* var. *quinckeanum*
(*Hughes* 1958)	*T. phaseoliforme*
Genus: Trichophyton	*T. rubrum*
Species: *T. ajelloi*	*T. schoenleinii*
T. concentricum	*T. simii*
T. equinum	*T. soudanense*
T. flavescens	*T. terrestre* complex
T. gallinae	*T. tonsurans*
T. georgiae	*T. vanbreuseghemii*
T. gloriae	*T. yaoundei*
T. gourvilii	*T. violaceum*

In the new classification adopted here, the imperfect fungi of medical importance, that were formerly classified in the order Pseudosaccharomycetales, are placed in the Class Blastomycetes of the Subdivision Deuteromycotina. These imperfect yeasts of medical importance are listed in table VI. It should be noted that four of the *Candida* species have a known perfect state classified in the Subdivision Ascomycotina and that one other yeast, *Cryptococcus neoformans*, has a perfect state referable to the Basidiomycotina (*Kwon-Chung*, 1975b).

The fungi formerly classified in the other four Orders (Sphaeropsidales, Melanconiales, Moniliales, Mycelia Sterila) are now treated in the Classes Hyphomycetes and Coelomycetes.

The majority of the fungus species that are capable of infecting humans and lower animals are found in the Class Hyphomycetes of the Deuteromycotina. In their treatment of the Hyphomycetes, *Kendrick and Carmichael* (1973) abandoned the traditional hierarchical division into orders and families. Instead, they chose four sets of characteristics that pertained to conidiogeny and the conidia themselves. These characteristics were used to define the genera and to organize them for identification purposes. The four sets of characters used were (1) the Saccardoan spore group, (2) conidial configuration, (3) conidial color and (4) type of conidiogenous cell. On this basis and with the admonition that "the species included in a form genus are related to each other by the form of their conidia and conidiogenous apparatus, but not necessarily by phylogeny", they compiled a complete annotated list of the generic names that have been proposed for the Hyphomycetes. *Kendrick and Carmichael*'s treatment of these fungi should be consulted to ascertain the current status of hyphomycete classification. Their evaluation of generic names is authoritative and should be taken into consideration by all who work with the so-called imperfect fungi. "Keylists" with illustrations are provided for the genera based on the four sets of criteria cited previously.

In table VII a list is presented of most of the genera and species of pathogenic fungi of the Class Hyphomycetes. The generic names used and the species cited reflect the latest taxonomic concepts regarding their validity.

Barron (1968) classified the hyphomycetes that have been isolated from soil on the basis of conidial ontogeny. Ten basic types of conidial development were defined and characterized: Aleuriosporae, Annelosporae, Arthrosporae, Blastosporae, Botryosporae, Meristem Arthrosporae, Meristem Blastosporae, Phialosporae, Porosporae and Sympodulosporae. These types are based essentially on the sections developed by *Hughes* (1953). *Barron* is well aware of the difficulties that the new system presents to those who try to use it. But study of his system and usage will lead to proficiency in the identification of unknown fungi.

According to *Barron*'s classification, the genera with geophilic pathogenic species are distributed as follows among his 10 sporotypes:

I. Aleuriosporae
   Chrysosporium, Histoplasma, Microsporum, Trichophyton
II. Annelosporae
   None
III. Arthrosporae
   Chrysosporium, Geotrichum, Trichosporon
IV. Blastosporae
   Candida, Cladosporium, Cryptococcus, Torulopsis, Trichosporon
V. Botryoblastosporae
   None
VI. Meristem Arthrosporae
   None
VII. Meristem Blastosporae
   None
VIII. Phialosporae
   Aspergillus, Fusarium, Penicillium, Phialophora
IX. Porosporae
   Curvularia, Drechslera, Torula
X. Sympodulosporae
   Dactylaria, Sporothrix

Table VIII. Genera and pathogenic species of the class Coelomycetes of the subdivision Deuteromycotina

Order: Sphaeropsidales	Genus: Phoma
Family[1]	Species: *P. hibernica*
Genus: Hendersonula	Genus: Pyrenochaeta
Species: *H. toruloidea*	Species: *P. romeroi*
(*Gentles and Evans* 1970)	*P. unguis-hominis*
	(*Punithalingham and English* 1975)

[1] *Sutton* (1973) does not divide the orders into families.

Recently, *Galgoczy* (1975) studied the conidial ontogeny of a group of dermatophytes. He found that they all were classifiable in *Hughes'* Section III, which corresponds to *Barron*'s Aleuriosporae.

The Class Coelomycetes accommodates a few fungi of medical importance. Those genera and species are cited in table VIII.

In this review, an attempt has been made to introduce the reader to the most recent developments in the taxonomic treatment of the fungi. Old concepts regarding the phylogenetic relationship of fungi to the algae and all other plants have been discarded. The fungi now reign in their own Kingdom. Other significant changes have occurred in the treatment of the imperfect fungi formerly classified in the Order Moniliales of the Class Deuteromycetes. The Saccardoan approach to their classification has been found unsatisfactory. In its place, a new system based on conidial ontogeny has been developed and adopted by modern mycologists. As a result of these fundamental changes, a large number of fungi of medical importance have been transferred to new genera, have had their validity as species denied, or have been found to merit variety status at best. The discovery of the perfect states of a number of pathogenic fungi has also led to their reclassification as ascomycetes or basidiomycetes.

In tables III–VIII, 140 species of fungi are classified. Of these, 27 have perfect as well as imperfect states and are cited twice – once under either the Ascomycotina or Basidiomycotina and once under the Deuteromycotina. This tabulation will be subject to change for several reasons. From time to time the validity of genera and species comes under question. Such taxonomic scrutiny frequently results in changes in nomenclature and classification. It should also be remembered that new species of fungi continue to be reported as infectious disease agents. This situation arises from the vulnerability of compromised hosts to infection by fungi previously not known to be pathogenic. These "opportunistic" fungi have a latent ability to develop in tissues once they have entered the body through inhalation or trauma. Individuals either suffering from chronic diseases, afflicted with immunological defects, under treatment with antibiotics or immunosuppressive drugs, or undergoing radiation therapy are the usual victims of these fungi which ordinarily would be dismissed as saprophytic contaminants in a diagnostic laboratory.

Medical mycologists must become acquainted with these changes and learn to appreciate the fact that taxonomy is in a continually evolving state of development. Tolerance and understanding is required as taxonomists strive to develop a classification system based on evolutionary theory and phylogenetic criteria.

References

Ainsworth, G.C.: Ainsworth and Bisby's Dictionary of the Fungi; 6th ed. (Commonwealth Mycol. Inst., Kew 1971).

Ainsworth, G.C.: Introduction and keys to higher taxa; in *Ainsworth, Sparrow* and *Sussman*, The Fungi, vol. IV A, chapter 1, pp. 1–7 (Academic Press, New York 1973).

Ajello, L.; Dean, D.F., and Irwin, R.S.: The zygomycete *Saksenaea vasiformis* as a pathogen of humans with a critical review of the etiology of zygomycosis. Mycologia 67: 1109–1113 (1975).

Arx, J.A. von: Testudinaceae, a new family of ascomycetes. Persoonia 6: 365–369 (1971).

Austwick, P.K.C. and Copland, J.W.: Swamp cancer. Nature, Lond. 250: 84 (1974).

Barron, G.L.: The genera of hyphomycetes from soil (Williams & Wilkins, Baltimore 1968).

Borelli, D.: El nombre correcto es Piedraia hortae. Derm. venezolana 1: 357 (1959).

Borelli, D.: Acrotheca aquaspersa nova species agente de cromonicosis. Acta cient. venezolana 23: 193–196 (1972).

Butler, E.E. and Petersen, L.J.: Endomyces geotrichum, a perfect state of *Geotrichum candidum.* Mycologia 64: 365–374 (1972).

Carmichael, J.W.: Chrysosporium and some aleuriosporic hyphomycetes. Can. J. Bot. 40: 1137–1173 (1962).

Carter, M.E.; Cordes, D.W.; de Menna, M.E., and Hunter, R.: Fungi isolated from bovine mycotic abortion and pneumonia with special reference to *Mortierella wolfii.* Res. vet. Sci. 14: 201–206 (1973).

Galgóczy, J.: Dermatophytes: conidium-ontogeny and classification. Acta microbiol. Acad. Sci. hung. 22: 105–136 (1975).

Gams, W.: Cephalosporium-artige Schimmelpilze (Hyphomycetes) (Fischer, Stuttgart 1971).

Gentles, J.C. and Evans, E.G.V.: Infection of the feet and nails with *Hendersonula toruloidea.* Sabouraudia 8: 72–75 (1970).

Hasegewa, A. and Usui, K.: In press (1976).

Hawksworth, D.L. and Booth, C: A revision of the genus *Zopfia* Rabenh. Mycological Papers. No. 135 (Commonwealth Mycological Institute, Kew 1974).

Hughes, S.J.: Conidiophores, conidia and classification. Can. J. Bot. 31: 560–576 (1953).

Hughes, S.J.: Revisiones hyphomycetum aliquot cum appendice de nominibus rejiciendis. Can. J. Bot. 36: 727–836 (1958).

Kendrick, W.B. and Carmichael, J.W.: Hyphomycetes; in *Ainsworth, Sparrow and Sussman* The Fungi, vol. IV B, chapter 10 (Academic Press, New York 1973).

Kligman, A.M.: A basidiomycete probably causing onychomycosis. J. Invest. Derm. 14: 67–70 (1950).

Kreger-van Rij, N.J.W.: Endomycetales, basidiomycetous yeasts, and related fungi; in *Ainsworth, Sparrow and Sussman* The Fungi, vol. IV A, chapter 2 (Academic Press, New York 1973).

Kwon-Chung, K.J.: Emmonsiella capsulata: Perfect state of *Histoplasma capsulatum.* Science *177:* 368–369 (1972).
Kwon-Chung, K.J.: Perfect state *(Emmonsiella capsulata)* of the fungus causing large-form African histoplasmosis. Mycologia *67:* 980–990 (1975a).
Kwon-Chung, K.J.: Description of a new genus *Filobasidiella,* the perfect state of *Cryptococcus neoformans.* Mycologia *67:* 1197–1200 (1975b).
Lodder, J.: The yeasts (North-Holland, Amsterdam 1970).
Malloch, D.: New concepts in the *Microascaceae* illustrated by two new species. Mycologia *62:* 727–740 (1970).
McDonough, D.W. and Lewis, A.L.: The ascigerous state of *Blastomyces dermatitidis.* Mycologia *60:* 76–83 (1968).
Moore, M.; Russel, W.O., and Sacks, E.: Chronic leptomeningitis and ependymitis caused by Ustilago, probably *Ustilago zea* (corn smut). Am. J. Path. *22:* 761–777 (1946).
Preininger, T.: Durch Maisbrand *(Ustilago maydis)* bedingte Dermatomykose. Arch. Derm. Syph. *176:* 109–113 (1937).
Punithalingham, E. and English, M.P.: Pyrenochaeta unguis-hominis sp.nov. on human toe nails. Trans. Br. Mycol. Soc. *64:* 539–542 (1975).
Restrepo, A.; Greer, D.L.; Bodledo, M.; Osario, O., and Mondragon, H.: Ulceration of the palate caused by a basidiomycete *Schizophylhem commune.* Sabouraudia *11:* 201–204 (1973).
Speller, D.C.E. and Mac Iver, A.G.: Endocarditis caused by a *Coprinus* species: A fungus of the toadstool group. J. med. Microbiol. *4:* 370–374 (1971).
Sutton, B.C.: Coelomycetes; in *Ainsworth, Sparrow and Sussman* The Fungi, vol. IV A, chapter 11, pp. 513–582 (Academic Press, New York 1973).
Whittaker, R.H.: New concepts of kingdoms of organisms. Science *163:* 150–160 (1969).

Dr. *L. Ajello,* Mycology Division, Center for Disease Control, Public Health Service, U.S. Department of Health, Education and Welfare, *Atlanta, GA 30333* (USA)

Discussion

Dr. *Pine:* Dr. *Ajello* has stated that *H. capsulatum* and *H. duboisii* are probably the same species but different varieties. But regardless of taxonomy, it should be pointed out that when *Kwon-Chung* crossed these two and obtained asci, the ascospores formed were sterile. It should also be emphasized that *H. duboisii* is essentially found only in Africa. Of millions of cases of histoplasmosis in the U.S.A. and throughout the world, only 1 case (in Japan) of *H. duboisii* has been found out of Africa. This strongly suggests a genetic restriction and hints that the two organisms are different species.

Dr. *Ajello:* Time will clarify this issue. Certainly the two entities are closely related serologically. All of the *"duboisii"* isolates are of one serotype and this serotype is indistinguishable from the 1,4 serotype of *H. capsulatum.* Morphologically the two cannot be distinguished from each other in their mycelial form.

Dr. *Paretsky:* Have *in vitro* DNA hybridizations been attempted, to establish systematic or taxonomic fungal interrelationships?

Dr. *Ajello:* Such studies are just beginning and should yield significant information.

Diagnosis of Systemic Mycoses

W. Kaplan

Center for Disease Control, Public Health Service, U.S. Department of Health, Education, and Welfare, Atlanta, Ga.

Introduction

The clinical features of systemic mycoses are extremely variable and closely simulate those of other diseases. Therefore, it is virtually impossible to establish an accurate diagnosis of systemic mycoses on clinical grounds alone, and laboratory tests are required. A variety of tests are available. They include: (1) direct microscopic examinations of clinical materials for the presence of the etiologic agents, (2) cultural examinations of specimens for the presence of the etiologic agents, and (3) immunologic tests for mycotic infections. In this paper the various diagnostic tests and procedures for collecting, submitting and processing clinical specimens for laboratory examination are discussed.

Collection and Submission of Specimens

The proper collection and handling of clinical specimens are key factors in establishing a correct diagnosis of a systemic mycosis. Because the primary site of most systematic mycoses is pulmonary, respiratory tract secretions or tissue taken at biopsy or autopsy are the types of specimens most often collected for mycological study. Sputum is the specimen most frequently submitted to the laboratory. If mycological examination of sputum is to be successful, this material must be properly collected and treated (*Haley,* 1964). 24-hour collections of sputum are generally unsatisfactory, because they usually contain large numbers of bacteria and saprophytic fungi. The most satisfactory sputum samples are single cough specimens. They should be collected in sterile glass containers and transported to the laboratory as soon as possible. The time of day at which a specimen is collected and the method of collecting it are important. A specimen collected before breakfast is preferred. A sample collected after a meal is also satisfactory, provided it does not contain food particles. The patient should be instructed to rinse the mouth thoroughly and to expel sputum from the lungs, not saliva or nasopharyngeal secretions. The patient who raises little or no sputum can be induced to produce it by inhaling a heated aerosol of 5% saline or another nontoxic reagent. In all instances of suspected pulmonary mycoses, multiple sputum specimens collected on successive mornings, or at 2- to 3-day intervals, should be obtained. If sputum is not adequate or the sample is otherwise unsatisfactory, bronchial or tracheal aspirates may be helpful. Miniature brushes may be inserted through a bronchoscope to obtain bronchial cells, which are then aspirated, or intrabronchial forceps used to obtain bits of tissue directly from lesions. Biopsies of scalene lymph nodes or direct lung biopsies through the chest wall are also of great value. Biopsy material should be placed in a sterile container and kept moist for transfer to the laboratory. Other types of clinical material of pulmonary origin, such as empyema fluid, cavitary aspirates, pus or material from abscesses or draining sinuses, are also of diagnostic value and should be collected if warranted.

Although most systemic mycoses are primarily pulmonary, they frequently disseminate to other parts of the body, including the skin. Therefore, extrapulmonary clinical materials, such as spinal fluid, bone marrow, blood (collected in an anticoagulant), urine, and exudates or biopsies taken from lesions in the skin or other organs may be diagnostically highly useful. All such specimens should be placed in sterile containers for transfer to the laboratory. Swab specimens are, as a rule, of little or no diagnostic value. If a swab must be used, one should collect as much specimen as possible. It is very important that in the case of a tissue sample, only a portion should by placed in a fixative for histological study; the remainder should be submitted fresh for cultural examination. All too often the entire tissue specimen is fixed, precluding cultural studies.

Clinical specimens should be examined as soon as possible after they are collected. This is particularly important if the specimens are likely to be contaminated. Specimens are often collected far from the diagnostic laboratory to which they must be shipped. In such cases, it is usually not advisable to ship clinical materials, particularly if they are contaminated, because contaminating organisms overgrow the culture, making the isolation of the etiologic agent more difficult, if not impossible. Furthermore, some fungi, particularly *Histoplasma capsulatum,* die out in clinical materials. For these reasons it is preferable to inoculate culture media and ship cultures instead of actual specimens for mycological study. Smears and fixed tissues can, of course, be shipped to distant laboratories.

If specimens must be shipped, steps should be taken to inhibit multiplication of contaminants (*Larsh and Goodman,* 1974). Antibiotics, such as penicillin (20 units/ml), streptomycin (40 units/ml), or chloramphenicol (0.05 mg/ml) can be added to the sample to prevent heavy bacterial growth.

Some antibacterial antibiotics, such as penicillin, inhibit *Nocardia sp.* and *Actinomyces sp.* and should not be added to specimens that are to be cultured for those organisms. Refrigeration of specimens during transport suppresses contaminants. Shipping frozen specimens is not recommended as a routine procedure, however, since some pathogenic fungi, particularly *H. capsulatum*, may not survive. Material obtained under sterile conditions and not considered to be contaminated, such as blood, bone marrow, spinal fluid and pus aspirated from closed lesions, may be shipped by mail, provided it has been collected in sterile, tightly sealed vials or tubes. Unfixed tissue can be placed in a small quantity of sterile saline and kept cool in transit. If tissue is contaminated, antibiotics can be added to the saline.

Specimens should not be stored in the laboratory before processing. If, however, they must be stored, or if they are to be stored for reference purposes, they should be kept in a refrigerator (4°C). Here also, antibiotics may be added to suppress the growth of bacterial contaminants. Storage in a freezer is not recommended, however, because some fungi, particularly *H. capsulatum*, may not survive freezing. In any case, storage should not be prolonged.

Processing of Specimens for Mycological Examinations

Many effective processing techniques are available. These procedures differ with the type of specimen, the test to be performed, and the particular diagnostic problem. The more common techniques for processing specimens are described below.

Cerebrospinal fluid and urine should first be centrifuged and a portion of the sediment cultured. Smears are prepared from this material for direct microscopic examination and, if required, for fluorescent antibody (FA) examination. The sediment is also examined as a wet mount and as an India ink preparation.

Pus and exudates are cultured. Smears are prepared for direct microscopic examinations and, if required, for FA examination. This material can also be examined as a wet mount and as an India ink preparation.

Tissue should be examined for purulent, caseous, or other types of lesions, and smears should be made of this material for direct microscopic examination, and, if required, for FA study. This material should also be cultured, and it can also be examined as wet mounts. If gross abnormalities are not evident, impression smears of cut surfaces of tissue should be made. A portion of the tissue should be fixed in 10% neutral formalin solution, or another fixative, for histological examination. The remainder of the tissue should be cut into small fragments with sterile scissors and forceps. The fragments may be cultured. However, it is preferable to grind the fragments in a Ten Broeck homogenizer or in a mortar and then to culture the homogenate. Smears of the ground tissue can also be prepared for direct microscopic examination and for FA study.

Blood and bone marrow specimens should be cultured and smears prepared for direct microscopic examination and, if required, for FA study.

Sputum and bronchial aspirates should be examined for blood and for purulent or caseous material. Such material should be cultured and examined as wet preparations. Smears can also be prepared for direct microscopic and FA examinations. The remaining specimen may then be concentrated by digestion and centrifugation, and the sediment examined microscopically and culturally. Concentration of the sample is not recommended for isolation of *H. capsulatum* when culture media are used, because centrifugation will concentrate the *Candida* sp. cells that may be present, and these frequently prevent the isolation of *H. capsulatum* (*Haley and Standard*, 1973). When laboratory animals are used for isolating *H. capsulatum*, concentration of the sample is advisable. Enzymes such as pancreatin or trypsin can be used. The chemical digestants N-acetyl-1-cysteine or dithiothreitol, however, are highly recommended for this purpose since they rapidly liquefy sputa. In most instances, samples can be digested in less than 1 minute. For such chemical digestion an equal volume of 0.5% solution of either reagent in 2.94% sodium citrate is added to the sputum sample (*Reep and Kaplan*, 1972). The mixture is gently agitated and, when the sample is liquefied, centrifuged. Smears are prepared from the concentrated sediment for direct microscopic and FA examinations. The sediment is also cultured. When media are used to isolate *H. capsulatum* from sputum, the specimen should be homogenized. This is done by adding 2–3 ml of brain heart infusion broth or saline to the specimen and drawing the material in and out with a pipette or syringe, or agitating the specimen with glass beads in a paint shaker (*Haley and Standard*, 1973).

Direct Microscopic Examinations

Direct microscopic examinations are invaluable in establishing a diagnosis of a systemic mycotic disease. They are rapid, simple to perform and may result in an immediate diagnosis, or at least an immediate presumptive diagnosis. Furthermore, they enable the laboratory worker to select the appropriate subsequent tests.

Wet mounts of processed specimens can be examined without further treatment for the presence of the characteristic tissue forms of the etiologic agents. If the specimen is viscous and dense, a drop of 10% KOH is added, and the preparation is then heated gently over a flame before being examined. Dried smears of clinical specimens may be examined as wet mounts by adding a drop of saline or 10% KOH and mixing the dried material with the liquid. Smears of clinical materials are stained by the Giemsa, Wright, Gram or modified Kinyoun's acid fast methods and examined for fungal elements and bacteria. Some laboratories use the periodic acid-Schiff (PAS) procedure for direct staining of smears. This stain is very effective in delineating fungi in smears of clinical specimens. For the detection of *Cryptococcus neoformans* India ink mounts are prepared and examined for the presence of encapsulated yeast cells.

The microscopic examination of stained tissue sections is an excellent method for diagnosing a mycotic infection. Histological studies enable the laboratory worker to detect the presence of fungal elements and establish tissue invasion, confirmation of which is of great diagnostic value in opportunistic fungal infections. Various histological stains can be employed. The hematoxylin and eosin (H & E) stain is very useful. Its advantages are that it permits observation of whether the fungus is hyaline or dematiaceous. The principal limitation of the H & E stain is that it does not stain some fungi and stains others poorly. Special fungus stains, such as the Gomori methenamine-silver nitrate (GMS), the Gridley, and the PAS, are superior to the H & E stain for delineating fungi. These histological stains are based on the principle that adjacent hydroxyl groups in the polysaccharides in fungal cell walls are oxidized, by using chromic or periodic acid, to aldehydes. The aldehydes are then stained with Schiff's reagent in the Gridley and PAS procedures. In the Gomori stain procedure, the aldehydes reduce the methenamine-silver nitrate complex, and the fungal cells are coated with reduced silver. Fungi stained by these methods stand out in sharp contrast to the surrounding tissue.

In general, the GMS method is better than the PAS or the Gridley method for screening. It stains the old and the nonviable fungus elements and filaments of *Actinomyces* and *Nocardia sp.* better than the other two stains. One limitation of the special fungus stains is that they do not allow one to determine whether the fungus is hyaline or dematiaceous. The GMS method stains all fungi black-brown. The PAS and Gridley procedures stain fungi a reddish color, which may mask the innate color of the organism. Another limitation is that the special stains do not allow the proper study of tissue response to fungus invasion. The combined H & E-Gomori procedure is useful in examining sections for the presence of fungi and for tissue reaction, especially if black and white photomicrographs are to be made of the material.

Mayer's mucicarmine stain can be used to differentiate *C. neoformans* from most other fungi of similar size and form. It stains the mucopolysaccharide in the capsular material of this fungus. It is not, however, specific for *C. neoformans* because it also stains *Blastomyces dermatitidis* and *Rhinosporidium seeberi*. The latter, however, is morphologically different from *C. neoformans* and can hardly be mistaken for it.

A Gram stain, such as the Brown and Brenn or the MacCallum-Goodpasture, is also very useful in histologic studies of mycotic infections. Although some fungi are stained by the Gram procedure, it is not generally recommended as a routine stain for fungi. It does stain *Actinomyces* and *Nocardia sp.* and can be used to detect these organisms. The Gram method is useful for identifying bacteria that may be causing a lesion under study or may be aggravating the fungus infection.

An acid-fast stain, such as the modified Kinyoun acid-fast, is useful in detecting *Nocardia asteroides, N. brasiliensis,* and *N. caviae.* The Manual of Histologic Staining Methods of the Armed Forces Institute of Pathology (1968) is valuable as a reference volume for histopathologic procedures and special stains for fungi.

A systemic mycosis can be diagnosed by direct microscopy with confidence, if the etiologic agent produces diagnostically distinct forms in tissue and if it is in its typical form. If such features are absent, the diagnosis is only presumptive. FA staining is very useful for detecting and identifying fungi in clinical materials (*Kaplan,* 1975). Because of the added dimension of serologic specificity, this stain can increase the accuracy of direct examinations. The FA technique can be used to detect and identify fungi in smears of most types of clinical materials and in sections of formalin-fixed, paraffin-embedded tissue. Smears can be fixed by heat or other fixatives. Paraffin sections can be deparaffinized in the usual manner by passage through two changes of xylol and then through graded concentrations of alcohol to buffered saline, pH 7.2. The direct application of FA reagents to deparaffinized sections may be satisfactory, if the sections have been cut thin (4–6 μm or less), if fungus elements are numerous, and if the tissue is not dense. These desirable conditions are not always encountered. Better results are obtained when deparaffinized sections are digested in 1.0% trypsin solution (pH 8.0) for 1 h at 37°C before FA reagents are applied.

The FA technique is useful in detecting and identifying fungi in histologic sections previously stained with H & E, or by the Giemsa, Brown and Brenn, or the Wright method. For FA staining of fungi in such previously stained sections, cover slips are removed by heating the slides to soften the adhesive and immersing them in xylol to remove the cover slips and residual adhesive. The preparations are then rinsed in phosphate-buffered saline, pH 7.2, and digested in 1.0% trypsin, pH 8.0, as are unstained, deparaffinized sections. Fungi in sections previously stained by the PAS, Gridley, or Gomori methanamine-silver nitrate procedures cannot, as a rule, be stained by the FA procedure. Apparently, the oxidation of polysaccharides in the walls of the fungi alters the antigenicity of the organisms so that they do not react with the labeled antibodies.

Prolonged storage of formalin-fixed tissues, either wet or in paraffin blocks, does not seem to affect the antigenicity of fungi. Therefore, the FA procedure can be used to diagnose a mycotic infection in retrospect and to diagnose a current infection. The antigenic stability of fungi makes possible the shipment of smears, as well as fixed tissues, to distant central laboratories for FA examinations.

The direct FA procedure is the one most commonly used for detecting and identifying fungi in clinical specimens (*Kaplan,* 1973). Sensitive and specific reagents have been developed for the detection and identification of *C. neoformans* and the tissue form of *B. dermatitidis, Coccidioides immitis,* and *Sporothrix schenckii.* A conjugate at first thought to be useful for the specific staining of the tissue form of *H. capsulatum* was produced by adsorbing fluorescein-labeled *H. capsulatum* antiglobulins with yeast-form cells of *B. dermatitidis.* Extensive evaluation disclosed, however, that this adsorbed reagent did not stain, or poorly stained, a number of *H. capsulatum* isolates. Most of these belonged to one of the five recognized serotypes of *H. capsulatum,* designated type 1,4. This deficiency severely limits this reagent's value for diagnostic purposes. A partially specific reagent prepared by adsorbing fluorescein-labeled *H. capsulatum* antiglobulins with *C. albicans* cells is preferable for diagnostic work (*Kaufman and Blumer,* 1968). This *C. albicans* — adsorbed reagent stains the yeast form of all known serotypes of *H. capsulatum,* and, with the exception of *B. dermatitidis* and *H. capsulatum* var. *duboisii,* apparently does not cross-stain other pathogenic fungi. Despite the presence of cross-reacting antibodies, this *C. albicans*-adsorbed product is very useful for diagnostic purposes. In most cases, the tissue form of *H. capsulatum* can be differentiated from that of *B. dermatitidis* on the basis of morphology. When required, these two fungi can be differentiated by FA procedures in which a conjugate specific for the tissue form of *B. dermatitidis* is used. The tissue form of *H. capsulatum* can be differentiated from that of the *H. capsulatum* var. *duboisii* by conventional methods. Reagents for demonstrating the tissue form of *Paracoccidioides brasiliensis* have also been developed; however, they need to be further evaluated. In contrast to progress in developing specific FA reagents for the tissue forms of the dimorphic fungi, relatively little progress has been made in producing specific reagents for their mycelial forms. Such reagents are not available. A number of investigators have attempted, without success, to produce specific reagents for the *Candida sp.* of medical importance. Some of the *Candida sp.* may be identified, however, by using a combination of adsorbed FA reagents. Furthermore, sensitive conjugates can be produced for differentiating members of the genus *Candida* of medical importance from morphologically similar heterologous organisms in clinical materials. Genus-specific conjugates for differentiating in-tissue aspergilli from morphologically similar fungi belonging to other genera have been produced. FA reagents, however, have not been produced for the differential identification of *Aspergillus sp.* Although protothecosis usually involves the skin in man, this disease usually appears in a systemic form in animals. Specific FA reagents have recently been developed for detecting and identifying the Prototheca species in culture and in formalin-fixed tissue (*Kaplan,* 1975).

The FA technique can be modified to measure and detect antibodies in sera and other body fluids. The indirect FA (IFA) procedure is generally used for this purpose. The IFA technique has been applied to detect antibodies to *C. neoformans*, *C. albicans*, and other *Candida sp.*, and to *Aspergillus sp.*, and it is used for this purpose in some medical mycologic centers. Another modification, the FA inhibition technique, has been found to be effective for detecting and measuring antibodies to *C. immitis* and for detecting antibodies to whole *H. capsulatum* yeast cells. Because other reliable serodiagnostic procedures are available for coccidioidomycosis and histoplasmosis, the FA inhibition test is not used routinely for the serological diagnosis of these two systemic mycoses.

Immunofluorescence has not yet received the widespread application that it merits. This deplorable situation stems in large part from the fact that very few FA reagents for the identification of fungi are available commercially. Fluorescein-labeled antiglobulins to *C. albicans* are on the market. More are needed, however, before FA procedures can be used routinely.

Cultural Examination

Cultural studies of clinical materials play a vital role in the diagnosis of systemic mycoses. When a basically pathogenic fungus is causing the disease, its isolation and identification constitutes a diagnosis. When an opportunistic fungus is involved, its recovery alone may not be sufficient to establish a definitive diagnosis. Evidence of tissue invasion is needed. Nevertheless, cultural studies are important in diagnosing opportunistic fungus diseases, because they enable the laboratory worker to identify the etiologic agent.

A variety of culture media are available for the isolation and identification of fungi (*Larsh*, 1970). Some contain antibiotics to inhibit contaminants. Some media are nutritionally lean; others are enriched. In suspected systemic mycoses, where the clinical findings do not point to a specific disease, it is generally advisable to use several types of media and to incubate cultures at both 25 and 37°C. The choice of media depends upon individual preference. The following isolation media are those used in the Mycology Division of the Center for Disease Control, Atlanta, Ga. (*Ajello et al.*, 1963): (1) Sabouraud dextrose agar; (2) Sabouraud dextrose agar with chloramphenicol (0.05 mg/ml) to inhibit bacterial contaminants; (3) Sabouraud dextrose agar with chloramphenicol (0.05 mg/ml) and cycloheximide (0.5 mg/ml) to inhibit bacterial and fungal contaminants; (4) brain heart infusion agar (or a similar enriched medium) with or without 6% blood; and (5) brain heart infusion agar with chloramphenicol (0.05 mg/ml) and cycloheximide (0.5 mg/ml). Specimens inoculated on the first three media are incubated at 25°C; those on the last two media are incubated at 37°C. Another very useful isolation media is Sabhi agar (*Gorman*, 1967), which is a combination of Sabouraud dextrose agar and brain heart infusion agar. Some workers have found that this combination of the two basic media is more effective for isolating pathogenic fungi than either of the two media used separately. Antibiotics can be incorporated in Sabhi agar. Specimens inoculated on Sabhi agar are incubated at 25°C. For safety, the use of slants is generally recommended. However, for cultural examinations of contaminated specimens, such as sputum, many workers prefer Petri dishes.

Some investigators (*Haley and Standard,* 1973) report that the millipore membrane filter technique is very useful in isolating pathogenic fungi; even small numbers of fungal elements are filtered from large-volume specimens. After the specimen is passed through the filter, the disc on which the fungal elements are collected is placed directly on solid culture media. If several isolation media are used, the disc is cut with sterile scissors and divided.

Safety precautions must be taken to prevent laboratory infections when systemic mycotic disease agents are being handled. Cultures should be handled under a biological safety hood to minimize the dissemination of infectious aerosols into a laboratory.

Many of the fungi that cause systemic disease can be identified on the basis of morphology. Special media and other substrates are available for inducing the production of diagnostic spores or other structures: for example, serum for inducing *C. albicans* to form germ-tubes and cornmeal agar with Tween 80 to induce it to form chlamydospores.

Accurate identification of the dimorphic fungi rests upon obtaining the two forms. Inoculation of laboratory animals is of great value in inducing the mycelial form of *C. immitis* to convert to the tissue form. Laboratory animals can also be used to convert the mycelial form of the other dimorphic fungi to the tissue form, but it is generally simpler to use artificial media for this purpose. Some mycelial-form cultures of *H. capsulatum* are very difficult, or sometimes impossible, to convert to the yeast form by conventional *in vitro* methods. Thus, the recent report by *Standard and Kaufman* (1976) on identifying mycelial-form cultures of *Histoplasma sp.* by immunodiffusion is of considerable interest to medical mycologists.

With few exceptions, the yeasts and yeast-like fungi cannot be definitively identified on the basis of morphology alone. Physiological tests, such as those which determine the fermentation and assimilation of sugars and nitrate, are needed. Standardized media and methods for carrying out the necessary physiological tests have been developed.

Laboratory animals are also useful for isolating pathogenic fungi, particularly from heavily contaminated specimens, such as sputum and environmental samples, or from specimens containing very few fungi. In such cases the animal's body serves as a primary isolation medium. Laboratory animals are useful in identifying fungi, as noted above. Pathogenicity tests, however, are not as widely used for the identification of fungi as they once were.

Immunodiagnostic Tests

Various immunodiagnostic tests have been developed for many of the systemic mycoses. Not only are they valuable diagnostic aids, they are also very useful in monitoring patient response to therapy and in predicting the course of illness. (For details, the reader is referred to Dr. *Kaufman's* paper.)

Concluding Comments

Fungal diseases constitute important public health problems. The systemic mycoses caused by pathogenic fungi are important primary diseases in many parts of the world. Furthermore, in recent years there has been a phenomenal increase in the incidence of systemic disease caused by opportunistic fungi that are essentially saprophytic. This increase stems from the widespread use of broad-spectrum antibiotics, immunosuppressants, and cytotoxic drugs to treat various diseases. Such opportunistic mycoses complicate treatment of the primary disease and may be the direct cause of death in the patient. Reliable laboratory methods are available for the diagnosis of all systemic mycoses. Both clinicians and laboratory workers should be aware that these diseases occur, and they should make use of these valuable diagnostic tests.

References

AFIP Manual of Histologic Staining Methods; 3rd ed. (McGraw-Hill, New York 1968).
Ajello, L.; Georg, L.K.; Kaplan, W., and Kaufman, L.: CDC Laboratory Manual for Medical Mycology. Public Health Service Publ. No. 994, Washington 1963.
Gorman, J.W.: Sabhi, a new culture medium for pathogenic fungi. Am. J. med. Technol. *33:* 151–157 (1967).
Haley, L.D.: Diagnostic medical mycology (Appleton-Century-Crofts, New York 1964).
Haley, L.D. and Standard, P.G.: Laboratory methods in medical mycology; 3rd ed. (Center for Disease Control, Public Health Service, US Department of Health, Education, and Welfare, Atlanta (1973).
Kaplan, W.: Direct fluorescent antibody tests for the diagnosis of mycotic diseases. Ann. clin. Lab. Sci. *3:* 25–29 (1973).
Kaplan, W.: Practical application of fluorescent antibody procedures in medical mycology. Proc. 3rd Int. Conf. Mycoses. Pan Am. Health Org. Sci. Publ. No. 304, pp. 178–185 (1975).
Kaufman, L. and Blumer, S.: Development and use of a polyvalent conjugate to differentiate *Histoplasma capsulatum* and *Histoplasma duboisii* from other pathogens. J. Bact. *95:* 1243–1246 (1968).
Larsh, H.W.: Isolation and identification media for systemic fungi. Proc. Int. Symp. Mycoses. Pan Amer. Health Org. Sci. Publ. No. 205, pp. 59–63 (1970).

Larsh, H.W. and Goodman, N.L.: Fungi of systemic mycoses; in Manual of clinical microbiology; 2nd ed., chapter 57, pp. 508–521 (Am. Soc. Microbiol. Washington 1974).

Reep, B.R. and Kaplan, W.: The use of N-acetyl-L-cysteine and dithiothreitol to process sputa for mycological and fluorescent antibody examinations. Hlth Lab. Sci. *9:* 118–124 (1972).

Standard, P.B. and Kaufman, L.: Specific immunologic test for the rapid identification of members of the genus *Histoplasma.* J. clin. Microbiol. *3:* 191–199 (1976).

Dr. *W. Kaplan,* Center for Disease Control, Public Health Service, US Department of Health, Education and Welfare, *Atlanta, GA 30333* (USA)

Discussion

Dr. *Austwick:* Is there any prospect of fluorescent anti-body staining reagents being made available more readily?

Dr. *Kaplan:* A few commercial firms have considered the possibility of producing and marketing such reagents. Indeed, Difco now sells fluorescein-labeled *C. albicans* antiglobulins. Sylvania Laboratories used to list fluorescein-labeled *C. albicans, S. schenkii* and *H. capsulatum* antiglobulins in their catalogue. They no longer do so. Whether in the future a broader use of FA reagents for fungi will be commercially available depends upon the market. There is a chance that market surveys will disclose that the market is large enough to warrant companies to produce such FA reagents.

In the meantime it is imperative that governmental agencies sponsor the production of FA reagents. WHO should support such programs.

In my opinion, FA reagents will be made more available in the future.

Experimental Infections with Fungi and Yeasts

D.B. Louria[1]

New Jersey Medical School, Newark, N.J.

Introduction

The goals of experiments in which fungi and yeasts are administered to experimental animals are varied, but can be categorized in the following general manner: (1) to determine organ predilection and the reasons therefore; (2) to analyze characteristics of the organism that promote pathogenicity or virulence; (3) to assess host defense mechanisms; (4) to analyze modifications in the host that either promote infection or alternatively aid the host to resist progressive multiplication; (5) to assess the comparative roles of microbial multiplication and microbial production of metabolites and toxins; (6) to measure host serologic response to invasion; (7) to determine the efficacy of antimicrobial agents either singly or in combination, with or without adjunctive substances. Most experimental design can be placed in at least one of the seven categories listed above.

The first question on which to focus is, which mycotic infections of major importance to man have been tested well enough that investigations have provided data relevant to the human condition in all or most of the categories listed above.

Obviously, there will be substantial diversity of opinion in regard to which fungi and yeasts can be considered as adequately investigated and which cannot. My own view is that the organisms studied most broadly are *Candida* species. Others in which the amount of information is extensive, but less complete, are *Histoplasma capsulatum*, *Cryptococcus neoformans* and *Coccidioides immitis*. Those for which the data are limited but still substantial include species of *Aspergillus*, the *Zygomycetes* (*Phycomycetes*) and *Blastomyces dermatitides*. Among

---

[1] The experimental studies cited in this paper were supported in part by NIH grant no. 1 R01 ES00888–03.

those fungi about which I feel there is inadequate information are *Sporotrix schenckii, Paracoccidiodes brasiliensis, Histoplasma capsulatum* var. *duboisii, Torulopsis glabrata* and those higher bacteria held to be in the purview of the mycologists, namely, *Actinomyces* species and *Nocardia asteroides*. In large part, lack of adequate information relates to failure to delineate a proper animal model.

I would like to discuss some of the experimental studies that appear to me to be of major interest with regard to the first three groups. I shall not attempt a comprehensive review, but will focus on our own data or on studies that seem to me to be particularly informative.

I. Candida albicans *and other* Candida *species*

The kidney appears to be the tissue most susceptible to progressive multiplication of this yeast in man (*Louria et al.*, 1962). The other organs frequently involved are the myocardium and the brain. This is precisely the situation in mice after intravenous inoculation of *C. albicans, C. tropicalis* or *C. stellatoidea* (*Louria et al.*, 1960, 1966; *Hurley*, 1966; *Hasenclever and Mitchell*, 1961). The finding in some series of human cases that the lungs are extensively involved (*Bodey*, 1966) needs clarification. In man, the lungs are often involved through hematogenous spread and consequent to this, perivascular foci of infection appear; but these are self-limited and only rarely result in extensive enough involvement that the lesions are visible on roentgenographic study.

The susceptibility of the kidney to progressive multiplication of this mycotic agent has been defined in reasonably satisfactory fashion (*Louria et al.*, 1960, 1966). After intravenous infection, the blastospores arrive in the kidney capillaries and once there, by presently undefined mechanisms, leave the capillaries, and gain access to the interstitial tissues where they are associated with a vigorous polymorphonuclear leukocyte response. That there is a rapid polymorphonuclear leukocyte (PMN) response seems clear, but the specific role and activity of the polymorphs are currently not certain. *Candida* cells are readily phagocytosed, at least by human and rabbit polymorphonuclear leukocytes (*Venkataraman et al.*, 1973; *Louria and Brayton*, 1964), but their fate thereafter is in dispute. We reported initially that blastospores survived after 4 hours' residence within human polymorphonuclear leukocytes. These studies were carried out by adding *Candida* cells to human peripheral polymorphs (PMNs) in a 2:1 blastospore to cell ratio, incubating the *Candida*-cell mixture at 37°C in a rotating apparatus and studying cell viability and phagoctosis by trypan blue staining with direct observation using a phase contrast lens. Survival was determined by pour plate enumeration techniques at 0 and 4 hours. This is a relatively crude bioassay; a 50 percent killing could not be detected by this technique in which $5 \times 10^6 - 10^7$ organisms were added per ml of human blood. *Lehrer and Cline* (1969a) did more precise studies using methylene-blue staining to determine the viability of *Candida cells*. They found approximately 30 percent of cells were killed by PMNs. In their experimental system, as in ours, a majority of cells survived. More recently, *Lehrer* has shown that killing occurs as the result of both myeloperoxidase-dependent and myeloperoxidase-independent systems (*Lehrer and Cline*, 1969b; *Lehrer*, 1972). Using *Lehrer*'s techniques, we found about 15 percent killing by rabbit or human PMNs, a finding very similar to that of *Laforce et al.* (1975). Perhaps the most relevant studies are those of *Davies and Denning* (1972). They took special precautions to maintain the viability of the leukocytes and added a very small inoculum, 200 blastospores per ml. Under these conditions, approximately 70 percent of *Candida* blastospores were killed within polymorphonuclear leukocytes.

Presumably, *Davies and Denning*'s (1972) study better imitates the ratio of *Candida* cells to host defense cells in clinical situations than our studies in which gigantic numbers of *Candida* cells were used. Consequently, it seems likely that the polymorphonuclear leukocyte response elicited by *Candida* tissue invasion does indeed reduce the numbers of invading organisms. This response is probably triggered by the chemotaxis resulting from a *Candida*-cell-wall mannan-complement complex (*Denning and Davies*, 1973). Some support for the notion that polymorphs are effective derives from observations that the interstitial abscesses in mouse tissues other than the kidneys are generally associated with control of the infection. Furthermore, it appears polymorphs can kill *Candida* even if phagocytosis does not take place (*Davies and Denning*, 1972).

In the kidneys, the situation is different. Within a few hours after interstitial invasion, the blastospores elongate, and these elongated yeasts rupture into both cortical and medullary tubules. They carry with them polymorphonuclear cells which rapidly become karyorrhectic and pyknotic. Thereafter, there is no additional leukocyte response within the tubular lumen. The elongated yeasts, having found a protected site for growth, now unimpeded by host cellular defenses, form mycelia that fill the tubular lumen. These mycelial elements then re-rupture into the renal parenchyma. The long mycelial elements are not now readily phagocytosed by host cellular defenses and form the nidus for large cortical and medullary abscesses.

Hurley and Winner (1961) have demonstrated that if the inoculum is not overwhelming, subacute and chronic renal lesions develop; these are characterized by collections of yeasts and mycelia in the renal tubules.

It seems clear that germ tube and mycelial formation is needed for pathogenicity (*Arai and Mikami*, 1975; *Young*, 1958; *Gresham and Whittle*, 1961). Strains that have lost or possess little of this ability cannot cause progressive disease (*Arai and Mikami*, 1975; *Gresham and Whittle*, 1961). The capacity to produce progressive renal infection in the mouse is shared by *C. albicans*, *C.*

stellatoidea and *C. tropicalis* but not by those species that have no capacity to form germ tubes and mycelia (*Goldstein et al.,* 1965).

The polymorphonuclear cell is not the only one able to ingest *Candida* cells. This is true also for alveolar macrophages of the rabbit which seem able to phagocytose but not kill the ingested yeasts (*Damodaran and Chakravarty,* 1973).

There may be additional factors accounting for growth in the kidneys; homogenates of kidney support growth of *C. albicans* better than homogenates of other tissues (*Mackenzie,* 1965). Although there appears to be ample explanation for the susceptibility of the kidneys to progressive multiplication of *C. albicans,* there is no such clear explanation for the localization of *Candida* abscesses in the heart and brain. However, brain homogenates, like kidney homogenates, appear particularly able to support *Candida* growth (*Mackenzie,* 1965).

Thus, the first two questions posed at the beginning of this essay seem relatively well-answered; germ tube formation by the organism and the protected environment of the renal tubular lumen account for tissue localization and much of the pathogenicity. This seems to apply to virtually all the species in which host-parasite relationships have been studied, including mice, rabbits, guinea pigs and man. The host defense mechanisms can be best understood by experiments that either augment or vitiate naturally occurring host defenses. The agents most used are adrenal glucocorticoids. Perhaps the most revealing studies carried out with steroids are those of *Hurley et al.* (1975). They chose the guinea pig because this species is somewhat resistant to the effects of corticosteroids and is similar to man in this respect. They found that long-acting steroids augmented infection, but they could not demonstrate abnormalities in either humoral immunity or the development of delayed immunity. Subsequent studies by the same group, using immunosuppressive agents, did not show striking enhancement of infection (*Hurley et al.,* 1975b), suggesting that steroid administration did not augment infection primarily by interfering with delayed immune mechanisms. It seems most likely that steroid effects relate in large part to delay in polymorphonuclear leukocyte mobilization. Unexplained is the fact that in immune guinea pigs, cortisone ablated the immune response (*Hurley et al.,* 1975a). This suggests that immune mononuclear cells play an important role, and two additional pieces of evidence suggest this is probably so. First, *Stanley and Hurley* (1969) and *Winner* (1975) found that mouse peritoneal cells do not control *C. albicans* or *C. tropicalis,* but if mice are first immunized, intracellular growth of *Candida* cells is strikingly reduced.

Second, we have carried out studies on mice using lead that strongly suggest that immune mononuclear cells are importantly involved. Mice were given lead acetate (10 to 200 mg/kg daily by force-feeding) or were injected subcutaneously or intraperitoneally daily with 100–300 μg of lead nitrate for 2 weeks prior to intravenous infection with 10^5 cells of *C. albicans.* At 2, 4, and 7 days, and at 2, 3, 4, 5, 6 and 7 weeks thereafter, liver and kidneys of 5 lead-treated

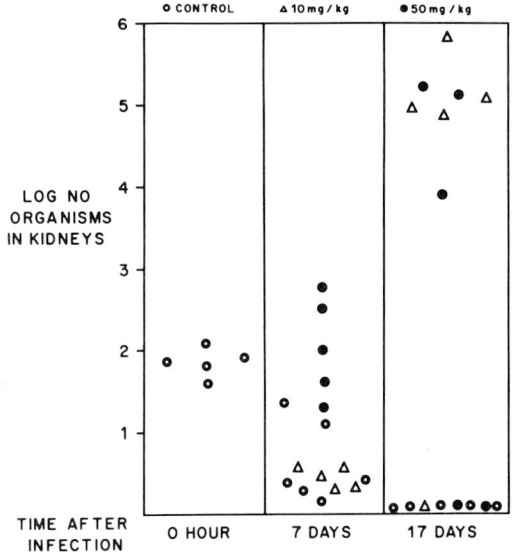

Fig. 1. Effect of lead acetate, 10 or 50 mg/kg daily orally, on intravenous *Candida* challenge.

and 5 control animals were removed aseptically, ground in a Vertis tissue homogenizer and viable *Candida* cells counted by making pour plates of serial 100-fold dilutions of the homogenate.

Two typical experiments are illustrated in figures 1 and 2. In figure 1, there is clear evidence of augmented multiplication in the kidneys, whereas in figure 2, there is delayed tissue clearance, but no evidence of augmented multiplication. Of interest is the observation that the modification of infection, either increased multiplication or delayed clearance, occurs after the first week and often not until the third or fourth week of infection. There is no evidence of an increase in the severity of infection during the initial 7 days after intravenously induced infection, the period when polymorphonuclear leukocytes are most involved. If it is not the polymorphonuclear leukocytes that are impaired, then presumably the augmented infection is related to interference with the function of the mononuclear phagocyte. There are, of course, alternative explanations. The lead may reduce the production of specific antibody that coats yeast cells and makes them more susceptible to either phagocytosis or intracellular killing by polymorphs. Lead is known to reduce the levels of circulating antibody (*Koller*, 1973). However, *Candida* cells are readily phagocytosed by human or rabbit polymorphs in the absence of immunization and can be seen within mouse polymorphs in tissues 4 hours after initiation of infection (*Louria et al.*, 1960).

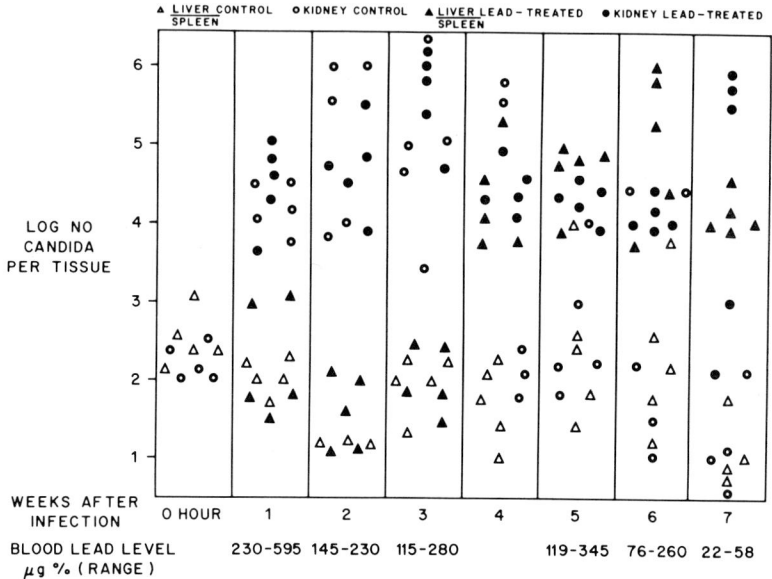

Fig. 2. Effect of lead nitrate, 5 mg/kg/day i.p., on intravenous *C. albicans* challenge.

Table I. Effects of lead nitrate, 10 mg/kg/day s.c. on macrophage clearance of staphylococci in mouse peritoneum

	Populations at		
	0 h	1 h[1]	
		lead-treated	control
Experiment 1			
	1.2×10^6	5×10^6	1.2×10^5
	5×10^5	6×10^5	3×10^4
	3×10^5	2×10^5	2×10^4
Experiment 2			
	7×10^7	3×10^7	2×10^7
	2.4×10^7	7×10^6	4×10^5
	1.5×10^7	10^6	6×10^4

[1] At the 1-hour period after infection, over 90% of cells in the peritoneal cavity are mononuclear.

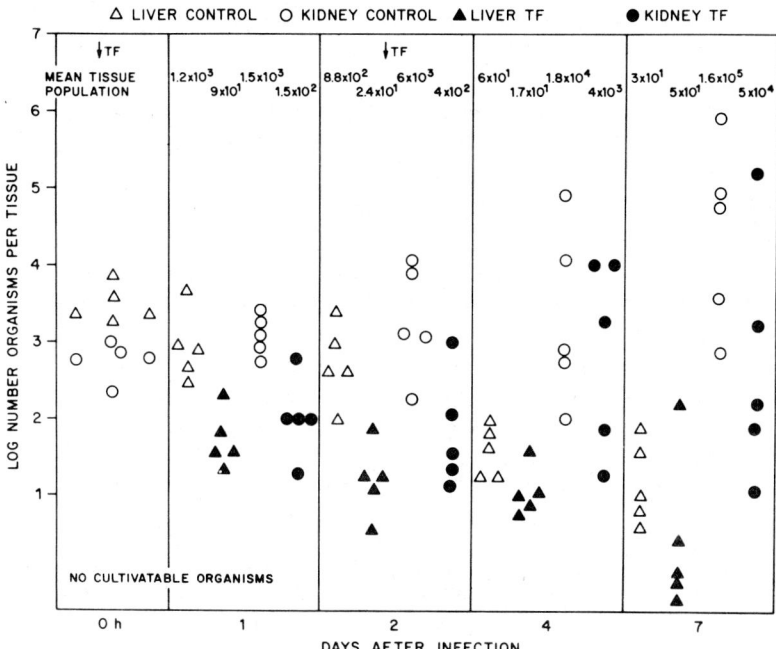

Fig. 3. Influence of transfer factor (TF) on intravenous challenge with 10^5 *C. albicans* cells in mice.

It is also possible that the effects observed relate in part to the nitrate or acetate rather than the lead. However, even if the acetate or nitrate are implicated, the point remains that late events are modified and that enhancement of multiplication is probably due to mononuclear rather than polymorphonuclear modification. Added weight for this supposition is found in observations (table I) that the administration of lead reduces the ability of mouse peritoneal macrophages to ingest and kill staphylococci during a 1-hour period after i.p. injection of the organism. Additionally, lead administration to guinea pigs appears in preliminary studies to interfere with skin test reactivity following administration of BCG.

The relative roles of the mononuclear phagocyte and leukocyte mobilization may be delineated by studies currently in progress on the influence of human transfer factor on experimental mouse candidosis. We have found that administration of $5 \times 10^6 - 10^7$ leukocyte equivalents to mice, either subcutaneously or intraperitoneally, modifies *Candida* tissue populations for a period of 1 to 2 days (and occasionally longer) (fig. 3). The modification occurs after administration of transfer factors from both *Candida* skin test positive and skin test negative human donors. The effects are therefore presumably non-specific and do not imply the transfer of specific immunologic information. Preliminary studies do not show any influence of transfer factor on mobilization of polymorphonuclear cells into the peritoneum after intraperitoneal injection of living or dead *Candida* cells. This suggests that augmented chemotaxis is not of major importance since chemotaxis is a major component in leukocyte mobilization into a tissue invaded by microorganisms. (Transfer factor does have potent chemotactic activity in other models) (*Gallin and Kirkpatrick*, 1974).

It may well be that transfer factor acts primarily by stimulating monocytes and that this stimulation augments macrophage anti-*Candida* activities. Another way of investigating the role of the mononuclear cell in disseminated candidosis would be to assess the effects of the T-cell-stimulating agent Levamisole on tissue populations.

There has been recent interest in 3 forms of localized candidosis. Hollingsworth and Carr (1973) injected rabbits intra-articularly with *C. albicans* and found that effusions did not develop for 2 weeks, reached a maximum at 3—4 weeks, and subsided 4 weeks later. Interestingly, cultures were negative at the time of maximum effusion. This model is probably more helpful in understanding the genesis of immune arthritis than in understanding *Candida* pathogenicity and virulence.

Recently, a technique has been developed for damaging heart valves and providing a setting for induced endocardial infection. For the most part, these infections have been bacterial and the model has been used to assess the effects of antimicrobials either singly or in combination. *Candida* infection has been initiated with this model (*Freedman and Johnson*, 1972), but here too, the major focus has been on therapy (*Bowman and Sande*, 1975). In both studies, blood cultures remained negative in most animals despite florid endocarditis. Similarly, splenomegaly was not found even at the height of infection (*Freedman and Johnson*, 1972).

Edwards and colleagues have established a model in rabbits for hematogenous *Candida* ophthalmitis. *C. albicans* infected the chorioretina and vitreous body, whereas *C. stellatoidea* and *C. tropicalis* showed far less ability to induce eye infection after intravenous inoculation (*Edwards et al.*, 1975, 1976).

One still inadequately answered question is the influence of *Candida* toxins. Hasenclever found that injection of large numbers of *Candida* cells into mice resulted in death during the first 12 hours, prior to evidence of microbial multiplication (*Hasenclever and Mitchell*, 1962). Salvin (1952) reported that intraperitoneal injection of mice with dead yeasts plus adjuvant was lethal. The role of *Candida* toxins has evoked increased interest recently, but it is still unclear whether toxins are of major importance in *Candida* invasion, either in man or experimental animals.

Mouse models have also been useful in assessing immunity in *Candida* infections (*Mourad and Friedman*, 1961; *Soles et al.*, 1967; *Saunders et al.*, 1975; *Dobias*, 1969). Heat-killed *Candida* affords very little protection, but living cells at a non-lethal dosage do increase resistance of the mice to subsequent ordinarily lethal challenge (*Mourad and Friedman*, 1961; *Soles et al.*, 1967). Equal protection can be induced by cell wall preparations (*Dobias*, 1964). The most impressive recent studies have shown that ribosomal preparations of *C. albicans*, if combined with *Freund*'s incomplete adjuvant, produce striking protection against lethal challenge (*Saunders et al.*, 1975). The use of ribosomal preparations alone, (without *Freund*'s incomplete adjuvant) induced a lesser protective effect. The precise mechanisms underlying the protection are not yet elucidated. There is no reason to believe that protection depends on circulating antibody.

II. Histoplasma capsulatum, Cryptococcus neoformans and Coccidioides immitis

Procknow et al. (1960) infected mice intranasally with tuberculate chlamydospores of *H. capsulatum*. Within 36 hours, yeasts proliferated from the spores and then disseminated to other reticuloendothelial cells. It appeared that change from spores to invasive yeasts probably took place both extracellularly and intracellularly in mononuclear phagocytes. After intravenous injection, the organism resides within mononuclear cells and this results in marked hepatosplenomegaly in species such as the mouse. *H. capsulatum* is ingested by both polymorphonuclear leukocytes and mononuclear phagocytes, but is killed more effectively by the former (*Howard*, 1975). Initially, it appeared that generation time within macrophages did not differ in mononuclear cells from non-immune and immune mice (*Howard*, 1965). Subsequent studies using freshly harvested peritoneal macrophages showed that immune cells did limit intracellular growth (*Wu and Marcus*, 1963). *Howard et al.* (1971) performed meticulous studies which indicated that the immune mononuclear phagocytes did indeed limit the growth of *H. capsulatum* and did so under the direction of immune lymphocytes. This conclusion makes sense. Histoplasmosis, like tuberculosis or listeriosis, is an infection characterized by survival of the invading organism within mononuclear cells, and in such infections, control depends on immunity conferred by sensitized lymphocytes transmitting information to monocytes (and the monocyte-derived cells, the macrophages). The precise mechanisms of transmission of information is not clear. *Tripathy and Mackaness* in a series of elegant experiments showed clearly that control of *Listeria monocytogenes* infection in the mouse can be ablated by interfering with the lymphocyte phase of the immune response (*Tripathy and Mackaness*, 1969a, b). Similarly, the administration of antilymphocyte serum or cyclophosphamide enhanced *Histoplasma* infections in mice (*Adamson and Cozad*, 1969; *Cozad and Lindsey*, 1974; *Howard*, 1973). However, these observations do not prove that enhancement is due to interference solely with lymphocytes. Cyclophosphamide also alters circulating immunoglobulins and antilymphocyte serum appears to have broader activities than the mere suppression of lymphocytes. *Howard* (1973) also showed clearly that immunity and intracellular killing are at least to some extent disparate phenomena. Immune macrophages limit intracellular growth but do not kill a substantial proportion of the ingested *H. capsulatum* cells. Based on these observations, *Howard* (1973) suggests that control of *Histoplasma* infection depends upon continued suppression of intracellular growth by the lymphocyte-macrophage system rather than direct killing of the organisms. The observations are consistent with other studies. If small doses of *H. capsulatum* cells are inoculated into mice intravenously, populations increase and then, depending on strain and dose, will decrease in some animals, presumably following the appearance of immune lymphocytes and macrophages (*Rowley and Hubner*, 1956; *Salvin*, 1955). If a larger inoculum is used, lethal infection may ensue but the administration of sulfonamides, agents not particularly effective against *H. capsulatum*, will increase the survival rate of the animals, presumably by keeping invading organisms from overwhelming the defense system and allowing the delayed immune mechanisms of the animal to become operative and effective (*Louria and Feder*, 1957).

For the last two decades, there has been growing interest in immunization in histoplasmosis. Inoculation with heat-killed cells confers substantially less protection than inoculation of living yeast cells (*Bauman and Chick*, 1969). Until recently, there was increasing concentration on cell wall constituents as immunogens (*Garcia and Howard*, 1971), but studies by *Fiet and Tewari* (1974) show that excellent protection can be induced by the use of ribosomal vaccines. At present, the precise mechanisms are undefined, but presumably, cell wall or ribosomal constituents activate the lymphocyte-macrophage system. The superiority of living to killed whole cells as immunizing vehicles is consistent with the observations of *Howard* (1973), suggesting that continued antigenic stimulation is needed to keep the lymphocyte-macrophage system activated, thereby delaying intracellular generation times for subsequently invading microorganisms.

Coccidioidomycosis is extensively discussed in a separate paper in this volume and will not be further analysed here.

An enormous amount of information has been gathered in recent years with regard to experimental cryptococcal infections. It used to be thought that there were no adequate host defenses against *C. neoformans*, that progressive infection always occurred after intravenous inoculation of highly encapsulated strains and that there was a particular affinity for the brain, perhaps based on the availability in the brain of nutrients in concentrations ideal for maximal growth of the cryptococcal capsule.

We found that following injection of small numbers of highly encapsulated *C. neoformans* organisms into mice, progressive multiplication occurred for 4 weeks in all tissues, including the brain (*Louria et al.*, 1963). Thereafter, one-half of the mice died with hydrocephalus, but in the other 50 percent, populations of the organisms fell progressively in all tissues studied, including the brain. When the survivors were challenged with an ordinarily lethal inoculum 3 months after the initial intravenous infection, the challenged mice showed a marked increase in survival rate when compared with the controls. There was no evidence that protection was mediated by circulating immunoglobulins.

Many recent studies have demonstrated that neutrophils can ingest cryptococci with small to moderate capsules and these polymorphs will kill the majority of ingested organisms (although a substantial minority survive intracellular residence (*Diamond et al.*, 1972; *Tacker et al.*, 1972). The large capsule interferes with phagocytosis as does circulating cryptococcal polysaccharide (*Bulmer and Sans,* 1968). Phagocytosis appears to depend on a combination of antibody, properidin, the classic and the alternate complement pathways (*Diamond et al.,* 1974). Mononuclear cells also phagocytose cryptococci, but intracellular killing appears to be less effective within the mononuclear phagocytes (*Diamond and Bennett,* 1973; *Bulmer and Tacker,* 1975; *Mitchell and Friedman,* 1972). Thus, *Bulmer and Tacker* (1975) instilled *C. neoformans* into the trachea of guinea pigs and found no reduction in lung populations during a 6-hour experimental period; guinea pig macrophages ingested but did not kill *C. neoformans* cells.

The cerebrospinal fluid of patients with cryptococcal meningitis appears to possess no opsonizing capacity *per se* but does restore the opsonizing capacity of adsorbed serum (*Diamond and Bennett,* 1973). These data support the concept that host defense mechanisms are not effective in the central nervous system. *Diamond* (1974) has also shown that cryptococci are killed by mononuclear cells (either monocytes or lymphocytes) in the absence of phagocytosis; in this system, antibody is needed for killing.

The collected data indicate that immunity is almost certainly related to the lymphocyte-macrophage system, but the role of phagocytosis by mononuclear phagocytes, and the role of extracellular killing in the presence of circulating antibody, are not yet fully elucidated.

Farmer and Komorowski (1973) studied the histologic reaction to small and large capsule strains after intraperitoneal or intracerebral inoculation. There was little inflammatory response to the large capsule strain, whereas the small capsule strain elicited a prompt exudative response with extensive phagocytosis. This is of great interest since *C. neoformans* in soil possesses a small capsule (*Farhi et al,* 1970; *Ishaq et al.,* 1968). It would appear that inhaled organisms are not highly encapsulated and that they should be well handled by host cellular defenses. Some believe these data suggest that infection occurs via the intestinal tract, not the lungs. However, it still seems likely that infection in man is via the aerosol route. If this is true, it will be interesting to attempt to define the variables that allow the small capsule strain to survive and change into the more troublesome and virulent large capsule strains *in vivo*.

III. Other Fungi

Young dogs have been suggested as advantageous for the experimental study of *Blastomyces dermatitides* infections, but thus far, only limited information has resulted, and it is not clear that the use of larger animals is really necessary (*Smith et al.*, 1975; *Ebert et al.*, 1971; *Turner et al*, 1971). Cozad (1975) has found that intravenous infection of mice with $10^3 - 5 \times 10^3$ cells gives a predictable pattern in which the lung is the tissue of maximal infection. The reasons for tissue localization are not evident at present, but it does appear that delayed immune mechanisms are important in control of the infection. *Spencer and Cozad* (1973) showed that mice given live blastomyces cells, or killed cells plus adjuvant, resisted lethal challenge and that this resistance coincided with the development of delayed hypersensitivity as measured by the foot pad test.

When conidia of *Aspergillus* species are injected into mice, the tissues of maximum involvement, according to histopathologic studies, are kidneys, heart and brain (*Scholer*, 1959; *Purnell*, 1974). Of interest is the fact that these are the same tissues most extensively involved after intravenous inoculation of *C. albicans*. Purnell (1974) has shown that strains of *Aspergillus nidulans* differ strikingly in virulence. The host response was similar to more and less virulent strains, but the former produced the more extensive lesions. When *Aspergillus* spores are administered by aerosol, the spores are actively phagocytosed by the *in situ* phagocytic cell, the pulmonary macrophage (*Lundborg and Holma*, 1972). *Epstein et al.* (1967) and *Merkow et al.* (1968) performed meticulous experiments and showed that phagocytosis by lung macrophages was followed by lysozomal degranulation mobilization of polymorphonuclear leukocytes and control of infection. If mice were treated with adrenal glucocorticoids, lysozomes were stabilized, spores germinated intracellularly, polymorphs were not mobilized, and the invading fungus proliferated. These studies are important because most patients developing disseminated aspergillosis have been treated with steroids and the studies of *Epstein et al.* (1967) define an interrelationship between the first cell line of defense, the macrophage, and the cell probably needed for control, the polymorphonuclear leukocyte. Interestingly, the infection in mice differs from that in humans in that in man there is no particular predilection for the heart, brain and kidneys.

Delay in mobilization of polymorphonuclear leukocytes is also important in zygomycoses (mucormycosis). *Sheldon and Bauer* (1958, 1960) showed that alloxan-induced diabetes in rabbits is associated with progression of induced infection with *Rhizopus oryzae* and with activation of previously existing quiescent local mucor infections. Progression of the infection was associated with failure of mast cells to degranulate.

Rhizopus rhizopodiformis spread markedly in rhesus monkeys given prednisolone (*Baker and Lineares*, 1974). In this model, the spread of infection was accompanied by a brisk polymorphonuclear leukocyte response. These experiments do not really differ from the rabbit experiments of *Sheldon and Bauer* (1958), in which the early events were investigated. In both rabbit and monkey models, delayed leukocyte mobilization may well be the common factor in enhancement of infection.

Sethi (1972) has developed an experimental model for disseminated sporotrichosis in mice. This may be of substantial value, since heretofore it appeared that this fungus would not grow in warm tissues. Studies showing that *Sporotrix schenckii* grows better in cool rather than warm environments *in vitro* and *in vivo* have considerable applicability to the cutaneous form of the disease, but are not relevant to disseminated sporotrichosis. *Sethi*'s model may permit further studies that will illuminate the pathogenesis of the systemic form of the disease.

Perhaps the most impressive aspect of experimental fungal infections is the increasing sophistication of the studies and the increased use of fungi and yeasts in experimental models for delineation of host defense mechanisms in both normal and immunized hosts.

References

Adamson, D.M. and Cozad, G.C.: Effect of antilymphocyte serum on animals experimentally infected with *Histoplasma capsulatum* or *Cryptococcus neoformans.* J. Bact. *100:* 1271–1276 (1969).

Arai, T. and Mikami, Y.: Some attributes of parasite and host *Candida* infection. Presented at VIIth Congr. Int. Soc. of Human and Animal Mycology, Tokyo, 1975.

Baker, R.D. and Lineares, G.: Prednisolone-induced mucormycosis in rhesus monkeys. Sabouraudia *12:* 75–80 (1974).

Bauman, D.S. and Chick, E.W.: Immunoprotection against extrapulmonary histoplasmosis in hamsters Am. Rev. resp. Dis. *100:* 82–85 (1969).

Bodey, G.P.: Fungal infections complicating acute leukemia. J. chron. Dis. *19:* 667–687 (1966).

Bowman, C.R. and Sande, M.A.: Therapy of experimental *Candida albicans* endocarditis. Presented at 15th Intersci. Conf. on Antimicrobial Agents and Chemotherapy, Washington 1975.

Bulmer, G.S. and Tacker, J.R.: Phagocytosis of *Cryptococcus neoformans* by alveolar macrophages. Infec. Immunity *11:* 73–79 (1975).

Bulmer, G.S. and Sans, M.D.: Cryptococcus neoformans. III. Inhibition of phagocytosis. J. Bact. *95:* 5–8 (1968).

Cozad, G.C.: Role of lymphocytes in mycotic infections; in *Hasegana* Proc. 1st Intersec. Congr. of IAMS, vol. 4, p. 19 (1975).

Cozad, C.D. and Lindsey, T.J.: Effect of cyclophosphamide on *Histoplasma capsulatum* infections in mice. Infec. Immunity. *9:* 261–265 (1974).

Damodaran, V.N. and Chakravarty, S.C.: Mechanisms of production of *Candida* lesions in rabbits. J. med. Micro. *6:* 287–292 (1973).

Davies, R.R. and Denning, T.J.V.: Candida albicans and the fungicidal activity of the blood. Sabouraudia *10:* 301–312 (1972).

Denning, T.J.V. and Davies, R.R.: Candida albicans and the chemotaxis of polymorphonuclear neutrophils. Sabouraudia *11:* 210–221 (1973).

Diamond, R.D.: Antibody-dependent killing of *Cryptococcus neoformans* by human peripheral blood mononuclear cells. Nature *247:* 148–150 (1974).

Diamond, R.D. and Bennett, J.E.: Growth of *Cryptococcus neoformans* within human macrophages *in vitro.* Infec. Immunity *7:* 231–236 (1973).

Diamond, R.D.; May, S.E.; Kane, M.A.; Frank, M.M., and Bennett, J.E.: The role of classical and alternate complement pathways in host defenses against *Cryptococcus neoformans* infection. J. Immun. *112:* 2260–2270 (1974).

Diamond, R.D.; Root, R.K., and Bennett, J.E.: Factors influencing killing of *Cryptoccus neoformans* by human leukocytes *in vitro.* J. infect. Dis. *125:* 367–376 (1972).

Dobias, B.: Specific and Non-specific immunity in *Candida* infections. Acta med. scand. *176:* suppl. 421 (1964).

Ebert, J.W.; Jones, V.; Jones, R.D.; Weeks, R.J., and Tosh F.E.: Experimental canine histoplasmosis and blastomycosis. Mycopath. Mycol. appl. *45:* 285–300 (1971).

Edwards, J.E., jr.; Montgomery, J.Z.; Foos, R.Y.; Shaw, V.K., and Guze, L.B.: Experimental hematogenous endophthalmitis caused by *Candida albicans.* J. infect. Dis. *131:* 649–657 (1975).

Edwards, J.E., jr.; Montgomery, J.Z.; Ishida, K.; Morrison, J.O., and Guze, L.G.: Experimental hematogenous *Candida albicans* endophthalmitis. II. Variation in species ocular pathogenicity. J. infect. Dis. (in press, 1976).

Epstein, S.M.; Verney, E.; Miale, T.D., and Sidransky, H.: Studies on the pathogenesis of experimental pulmonary aspergillosis. Am. J. Path. *51:* 769–784 (1967).

Farhi, F.; Bulmer, G.S., and Tacker, J.R.: Cryptococcus neoformans. The not so encapsulated yeast. Infec. Immunity *1:* 526–531 (1970).

Farmer, S.G. and Komorowski, R.A.: Histologic response to capsule-deficient *Cryptococcus neoformans.* Archs Path. *96:* 383–387 (1973).

Fiet, C. and Tewari, R.P.: Immunogenicity of ribosomal preparations from yeast cells of *Histoplasma capsulatum.* Infec. Immunity *10:* 1091–1097 (1974).

Freedman, L.R. and Johnson, M.L.: Experimental endocarditis. IV. Tricuspid and aortic valve infection with *Candida albicans* in rabbits. Yale J. Biol. Med. *45:* 163–175 (1972).

Gallin, J.I. and Kirkpatrick, C.H.: Chemotactic activity in dialyzable transfer factor. Proc. natn. Acad. Sci. USA *71:* 498–502 (1974).

Garcia, J.P. and Howard, D.H.: Characterization of antigens from the yeast phase of *Histoplasma capsulatum.* Infec. Immunity *4:* 116–125 (1971).

Goldstein, E.; Grieco, M.H.; Gindel, G., and Louria, D.B.: Studies on the pathogenesis of experimental *Candida parapsilosis* and *Candida guilliermondii* infections in mice. J. infect. Dis. *115:* 293–302 (1965).

Gresham, G.A. and Whittle, C.H.: Studies of invasive, mycelial form of *Candida albicans.* Sabouraudia *1:* 30–33 (1961).

Hasenclever, H.F. and Mitchell, W.O.: Pathogenicity of *C. albicans* and *C. tropicalis.* Sabouraudia *1:* 16–21 (1961).

Hasenclever, H.F. and Mitchell, W.O.: Toxicity of *Candida albicans.* Bact. Proc.: 67 (1962).

Hollingsworth, J.W. and Carr, J.: Experimental candidal arthritis in the rabbit. Sabouraudia *11:* 56–58 (1973).

Howard, D.H.: Intracellular growth of *Histoplasma capsulatum.* J. Bact. *89:* 518–523 (1965).

Howard, D.H.: Further studies on the inhibition of *Histoplasma capsulatum* within macrophages from immunized animals. Infec. Immunity *8:* 577–581 (1973).

Howard, D.A.: Fungicidal systems derived from phagocytic cells. Presented at VIIth Congr. Int. Soc. Human and Animal Mycology, Tokyo 1975.
Howard, D.H.; Otto, F., and Gupta, R.K.: Lymphocyte-mediated cellular immunity in histoplasmosis. Infec. Immunity *4:* 605–610 (1971).
Hurley, R.: Pathogenicity of the genus *Candida* in *Winner and Hurley* Symposium on *Candida:*Infections, p. 13 (Livingston, Edinburgh 1966).
Hurley, D.L.; Balow, J.E., and Fauci, A.S.: Experimental disseminated candidiasis. II. Administration of glucocorticoids, susceptibility to infection and immunity. J. infect. Dis. *132:* 393–398 (1975a).
Hurley, D.L.; Balow, J.E., and Fauci, A.S.: Experimental candidiasis. Effects of cytotoxic drugs on immunity and infection. Clin. Res. *23:* 306A (1975b).
Hurley, R. and Winner, H.I.: Experimental renal moniliasis in the mouse. J. Path. Bact. *86:* 75–82 (1961).
Ishaq, C.M.; Bulmer, G.S., and Felton, F.G.: An evaluation of various environmental factors affecting propagation of *Cryptococcus neoformans.* Mycopath. Mycol. appl. *35:* 81–90 (1968).
Koller, L.D.: Immunosuppression produced by lead, cadmium and mercury. Am. J. vet. Res. *34:* 1457–1458 (1973).
Laforce, F.M.; Mills, D.M.; Iverson, K.; Cousins, R., and Everett, E.D.: Inhibition of leukocyte candidacidal activity by serum from patients with disseminated candidiasis. J. Lab. clin. Med. *86:* 657–666 (1975).
Lehrer, R.I.: Functional aspects of a second mechanism of candidicidal activity by human neutrophils. J. clin. Invest. *51:* 2566–2572 (1972).
Lehrer, R.I. and Cline, M.J.: Interaction of *Candida albicans* with human leukocytes and serum. J. Bact. *98:* 996–1004 (1969a).
Lehrer, R.I. and Cline, M.J.: Leukocyte myeloperoxidase deficiency and disseminated candidiasis: The role of myeloperoxidase in resistance to *Candida* infection. J. clin. Invest. *48:* 1478–1488 (1969b).
Louria, D.B. and Brayton, R.G.: Behavior of *Candida* cells within leukocytes. Proc. Soc. exp. Biol. Med. *115:* 93–98 (1964).
Louria, D.B.; Buse, M.; Brayton, R.G., and Finkel, G.: The pathogenesis of *Candida tropicalis* infections in mice. Sabouraudia *5:* 14–25 (1966).
Louria, D.B. and Feder, N.: Sulfonamides in experimental histoplasmosis. Ant. Chemo. *7:* 471–476 (1957).
Louria, D.B.; Fallon, N., and Browne, H.G.: The influence of cortisone on experimental fungus infections in mice. J. clin. Invest. *39:* 1435–1449 (1960).
Louria, D.B.; Kaminski, T., and Finkel, G.: Further studies on immunity in experimental cryptococcosis. J. exp. Med. *117:* 509–520 (1963).
Louria, D.B.; Stiff, D., and Bennett, B.: Disseminated moniliasis in the adult. Medicine *41:* 307–337 (1962).
Lundborg, M. and Holma, B.: In vitro phagocytosis of fungal spores by rabbit lung macrophages. Sabouraudia *10:* 152–156 (1972).
Mackenzie, D.W.R.: Studies on the morphogenesis of *Candida albicans.* II. Growth in organ extract. Sabouraudia *4:* 126–130 (1965).
Merkow, L.; Pardo, M.; Epstein, S.M.; Verney, E., and Sidransky, H.: Lysozomal stability during phagocytosis of *Aspergillus flavus* spores by alveolar macrophages of cortisone-treated mice. Science *160:* 79–81 (1968).
Mitchell, T.G. and Friedman, L.: In vitro phagocytosis and intracellular fate of variously encapsulated strains of *Cryptococcus neoformans.* Infec. Immunity *5:* 491–498 (1972).

Mourad, S. and Friedman, L.: Active immunization of mice against *Candida albicans*. Proc. Soc. exp. Biol. Med. *106:* 570–572 (1961).

Procknow, J.J.; Page, M.I., and Loosli, C.G.: Early pathogenesis of experimental histoplasmosis. Archs Path. *69:* 413–426 (1960).

Purnell, D.M.: The histopathologic response of mice to *Aspergillus nidulans*. Comparison between genetically defined haploid and diploid strains of different virulence. Sabouraudia *12:* 95–104 (1974).

Rowley, D.A. and Hubner, M.: Growth of *Histoplasma capsulatum* in normal, superinfected and immunized mice. J. Immun. *77:* 15–23 (1956).

Salvin, S.B.: Endotoxin in pathogenic fungi. J. Immun. *69:* 89–99 (1952).

Salvin, S.B.: Resistance to reinfection in experimental histoplasmosis. J. Immun. *74:* 214–221 (1955).

Saunders, E.S.; Tewari, R.P., and Solotorovsky, M.: Immunogenicity of ribosomal preparations from *Candida albicans*. Presented at VIIth Congr. Int. Soc. for Human and Animal Mycology, Tokyo 1975.

Scholer, H.J.: Experimentelle Aspergillose der Maus (*Aspergillus fumigatus*) and ihre chemotherapeutische Beeinflussung. Schweiz. 2. Path. Bakt. *22:* 564–576 (1959).

Sethi, K.K.: Experimental sporotrichosis in the normal and modified host. Sabouraudia *10:* 66–73 (1972).

Sheldon, W.H. and Bauer, H.: Activation of quiescent mucormycotic granulomata in rabbits by induction of acute alloxan diabetes. J. exp. Med. *108:* 171–177 (1958).

Sheldon, W.H. and Bauer, H.: Tissue mast cells and acute inflammation in experimental cutaneous mucormycosis of normal, 48/80 treated and diabetic rats. J. exp. Med. *112:* 1069–1083 (1960).

Smith, C.D.; Furcolow, M.L., and Hulker, P.W.: Distribution of *Blastomyces dermatitides* in dogs with skin test and serologic results following airborne infection. Sabouraudia *13:* 192–199 (1975).

Soles, P.; Lim, L.Y., and Louria, D.B.: Active immunity in experimental candidiasis in mice. Sabouraudia *5:* 315–322 (1967).

Spencer, H.D. and Cozad, G.C.: Role of delayed hypersensitivity in blastomycosis of mice. Infec. Immunity *7:* 329–334 (1973).

Stanley, V.C. and Hurley, R.: The growth of *Candida* species in cultures of mouse peritoneal macrophages. J. Path. *97:* 357–366 (1969).

Tacker, J.R.; Farhi, F., and Bulmer, G.S.: Intracellular fate of *Cryptococcus neoformans*. Infec. Immunity *6:* 162–167 (1972).

Tripathy, S.P. and Mackaness, G.B.: The effect of cytotoxic agents on the passive transfer of cell-mediated immunity. J. exp. Med. *130:* 17–30 (1969a).

Tripathy, S.P. and Mackaness, G.B.: The effect of cytotoxic agents on the primary response to *Listeria monocytogenes*. J. exp. Med. *130:* 1–16 (1969b).

Turner, C.; Furcolow, M.L., and Smith, C.D.: Experimental histoplasmosis and blastomycosis in young pups. Sabouraudia *12:* 188–192 (1971).

Venkataraman, M.; Mohapatra, L.N., and Bhoyan, U.N.: I. Phagocytosis of *Candida albicans* by neutrophils. Sabouraudia *11:* 183–191 (1973).

Wu, W.G. and Marcus, S.: Humoral factors in cellular resistance. J. Immun. *91:* 313–322 (1963).

Winner, H.I.: Candidosis: in Chick, Balows and Furcolow Opportunistic fungal infections p. 149 (Thomas, Springfield 1975).

Young, G.: The process of invasion and persistence of *Candida albicans* injected intraperitoneally into mice. J. infect. Dis. *102:* 114–120 (1958).

Dr. *D.B. Louria,* New Jersey Medical School, *Newark, NJ 07103* (USA)

Discussion

Dr. *Levine:* How do you account for the activity of transfer factor from the "naive" donor? Can you conceive of a normal human adult immunologically naive with respect to *C. albicans*?

Dr. *Louria:* If the human donor has a negative skin test to *Candida* antigens, and if the patient's leukocytes cannot release migration inhibition factor in the presence of *Candida* antigen, then we assume that for our purposes the person is *Candida* naive and cannot pass immunologic information through transfer factor. The derivative assumption is that the effects of transfer factor in our animal model are non-specific. We are now testing the transfer of immunologic information from man to mouse but we believe the results will be negative and that we will find that human transfer factor acts by non-specifically stimulating mast monocytes.

Pathogenesis and Therapy of Cryptococcosis in Animal Experiments

F. Staib, S.K. Mishra[1], G. Grosse and Th. Abel

Robert Koch Institute (Federal Health Office) and Institute of Pathology, Auguste Victoria Hospital, Berlin, Germany

Introduction

Staib, Mishra and Grosse (1975) reported about a strain of *Cryptococcus neoformans* which could be recovered from the brain only of mice sacrificed 4 weeks after intraperitoneal inoculation, in contradistinction to the fatal involvement of all organs caused by another strain under identical conditions. These observations prompted us to undertake a wider study of the pathogenicity and related morphological and nutritional aspects of a rather large number of strains. Here, we attempt to summarize and correlate all the available data having a possible bearing on the pathogenesis and therapy of cryptococcosis.

Materials and Methods

Pathogenicity of 31 Strains of C. neoformans:

Inocula were prepared from 31 strains of *C. neoformans* grown on Sabouraud agar for 48 h at 26°C. Groups of 15 male albino mice (NMRI, weighing about 18 g) were inoculated i.p. with each of the test strains, using a uniform dose of ca. 2×10^7 cells contained in 1 ml of 0.85% saline/mouse. Batches of 5 mice from each of the 31 groups were killed at 2, 4 and 7 weeks after inoculation. Their internal organs – brain, heart, liver, lung, spleen and kidney – were examined for the presence of cryptococci, as were also those of animals which died during the 7-week period.

The gross and microscopic morphology of the 31 strains grown on Sabouraud dextrose agar (SDA) at 26°C was studied, with special reference to the texture and appearance of the colony, capsule size and the tendency to form pseudomycelium or hypha-like structures.

---

[1] Fellow of the Alexander von Humboldt Foundation, Federal Republic of Germany

Uremia and Ocular Cryptococcosis:

Prompted by our previous clinical and experimental observations (*Staib et al.,* 1976a) on uremia and cryptococcosis of the eye, the following study was undertaken: Each of a group of 100 albino mice (as described in the previous experiment) of the same age and sex were inoculated i.p. with about 2×10^7 cells of *C. neoformans*, strain W 2/A 94 (*Staib and Mishra,* 1975a, b). At three weeks, a uremia of short duration was induced in 50 of these mice by injecting 0.2 ml glycerine intramuscularly (*Thiel et al.* 1967; *Staib et al.,* 1976a). The high level of low-molecular weight nitrogenous substances in the peripheral blood was detectable by the auxanographic method described by *Staib* (1964) and *Staib et al.* (1976b). Ten of these mice were subjected to 2 more periods of induced uremia, each lasting 2–3 days, at intervals of one week. The remaining 50 mice served as controls.

Effect of Uric Acid on C. neoformans:

The known ability of *C. neoformans* to utilize low molecular-weight nitrogenous substances as their sole source of nitrogen (*Staib,* 1962b, 1963a, b, c), and the fact that such compounds are common metabolic endproducts of birds and mammals, especially the former, whose excreta are usually found to harbour the pathogen, stimulated interest in studying the effect of uric acid on *C. neoformans*. Urea, creatinine and creatin were also included for comparison. This study was performed using a solid medium described by *Staib* (1963a, b) for creatinine assimilation, containing 0.01% of the test substance as sole source of nitrogen. One drop (0.05 ml) of a suspension of the test strain was placed on one side of a Petri-dish containing the medium and the plate was tilted in such a manner that the inoculum could spread on its surface, forming a thick line passing through the centre. The plates were incubated at 26°C and the gross and microscopic appearance of the growth on different media were recorded at intervals.

Results

Pathogenicity of 31 Strains of C. neoformans:

The observations made and data obtained in this study are summarized in Table I. The origin of the 31 strains apparently had no significance insofar as their virulence for white mice was concerned.

a. *Strains found only in the brain:* Of the 31 strains tested in mice, 6 showed a tendency to survive in the brain only for a limited period, usually 4 weeks after i.p. inoculation. Four of these strains formed mucoid colonies on SDA at 26°C, had medium-sized capsules and frequently showed pseudomycelium or hypha formation. The colonies of the remaining two strains appeared dry and pasty; one had no distinct capsule but showed a tendency to form hyphae while the other was marked by the presence of a small capsule and no mycelium or hypha formation. These strains killed usually less than 5% of the animals and in only a few mice was there macroscopic involvement of the central nervous system (CNS). Although these six strains preferentially survived in the brain, they were often also isolated from other organs of animals killed after two weeks. Exceptionally, strain A 97 could be recovered only from the brain even at two weeks after inoculation.

Table I. Principal morphological features of 31 strains of *C. neoformans* tested for virulence in white mice after i.p. inoculation.

Organ involvement	Mortality	Number of strains	Common morphological features		
			Colony appearance	Capsule (*in vitro*)	Pseudomycelium/ hypha-formation
* Brain only	Low	4	Mucoid	Medium	Present
		1	Dry	Absent	Present
		1	Dry	Small	Absent
** Other organs but not brain	None	4	Mucoid	Big	Absent
		1	Mucoid	Small	Absent
** All organs including brain	High	6	Mucoid	Big	Absent
		5	Mucoid	Medium	Absent
		9	Dry	Absent	Absent

* Four weeks after inoculation
** Over-all picture

b. *Strains found in other organs but not in the brain:* In contrast, five strains of *Cryptococcus* could not be isolated from the brain of i.p. inoculated mice, throughout the 7 week observation period. These strains always formed mucoid colonies on SDA but never showed pseudomycelium or hypha-like structures. Four had large capsules, and the fifth a small but distinct one. None of the mice inoculated with these strains died or appeared sick. Three strains, including the one with the small capsule, showed no evidence of dissemination to organs other than the peritoneal (spleen, kidney and liver); cryptococci were not recovered from brain, lung or heart blood of any of the infected mice. However, the other two strains were occasionally isolated from the lung also.

c. *Strains found in all the organs:* Twenty strains of *C. neoformans* caused progressive involvement of all organs, including the brain. The mortality rate in these groups of mice was usually very high — three strains killed all the mice within 2–3 weeks. None of these strains showed any preference for any particular organ, but a common pathological feature was the enlargement of spleen and lungs, particularly in the case of nine non-encapsulated dry-colony forming strains. As shown in Table I, eleven of these twenty strains formed mucoid

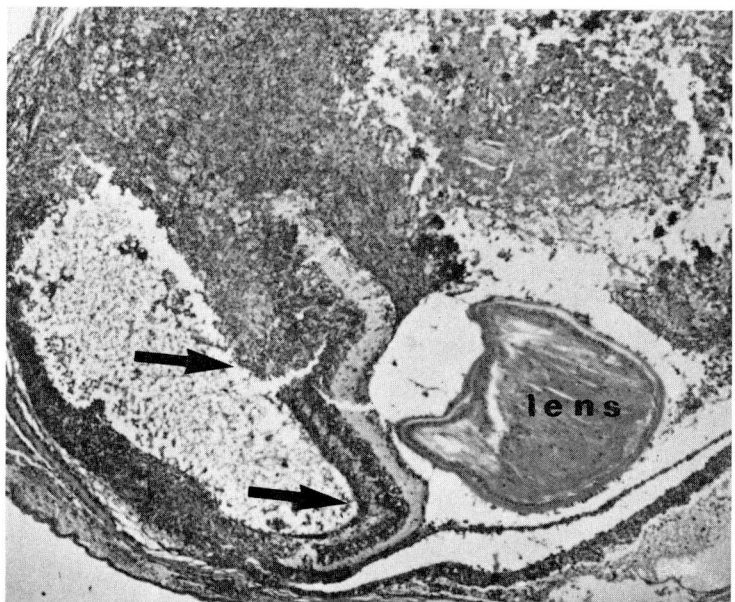

Fig. 1. Intraocular cryptococcosis in a uremic mouse killed 45 days after i.p. inoculation with *C. neoformans* strain W 2/A 94. The section shows panophthalmitis with detachment of the retina by the "cryptococcoma" (see the arrows), chorioretinitis and old abscess of the vitreous body. [Note the chronic granulomatous inflammation with foci of encapsulated cryptococci.] PAS stain, × 225

colonies on SDA; six of them had large capsules (ca. 3–4 μ), and the remaining five, medium sized ones (ca. 2 μ). None of these 20 strains showed any pseudomycelium or hypha formation of SDA at 26°C.

Uremia and Ocular Cryptococcosis:

Six weeks after i.p. inoculation, five uremic mice, including one which was subjected to three periods of uremia, began to show signs of involvement of one or both eyes, marked by blindness or grossly apparent turbidity of the eye and occasional proptosis. One of them died at this stage and the fungus was isolated from the eyes, brain and kidney. The other 4 mice appeared healthy, but when killed, the presence of the fungus in the brain was revealed. Normal as well as degenerated forms of cryptococci were detectable in the eyes of these mice on histopathological examination (Figs. 1–4). A process of spontaneous healing was also often seen. It was not always possible to isolate the fungus from the eyes of these animals. Three weeks later, three more mice, including two which suffered one period of uremia and one control, started showing signs of eye involvement,

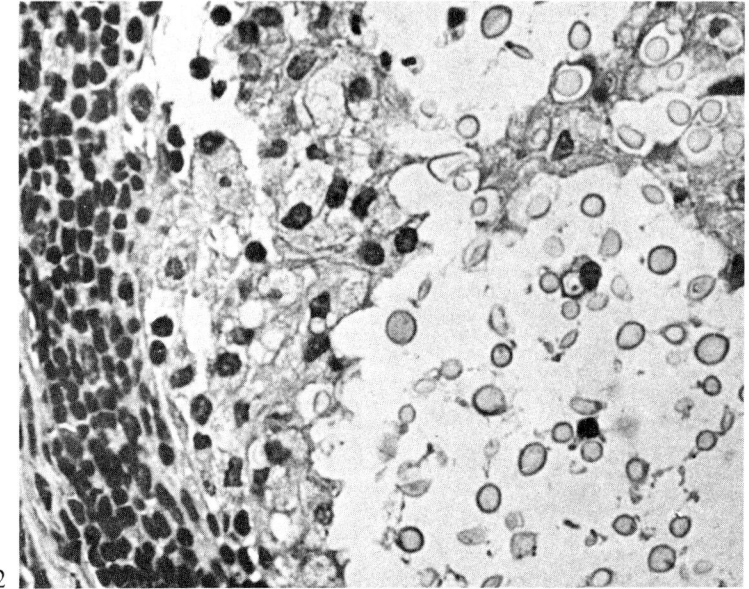

2

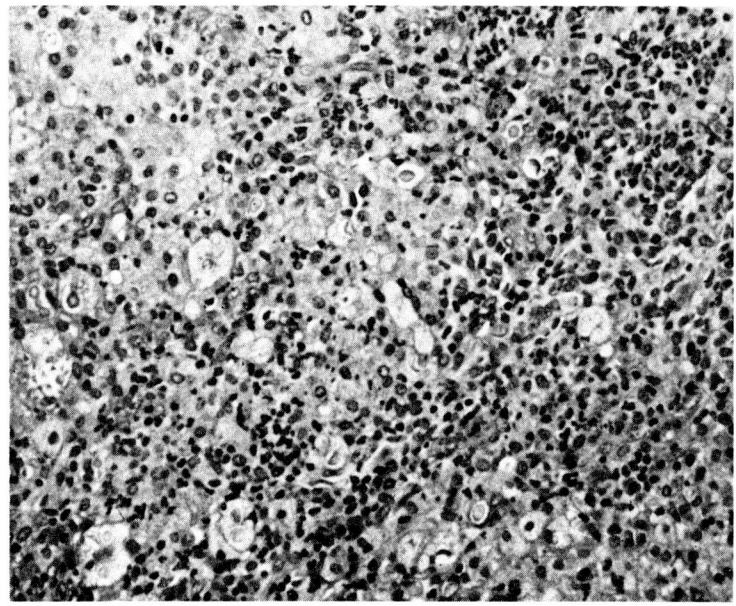

3

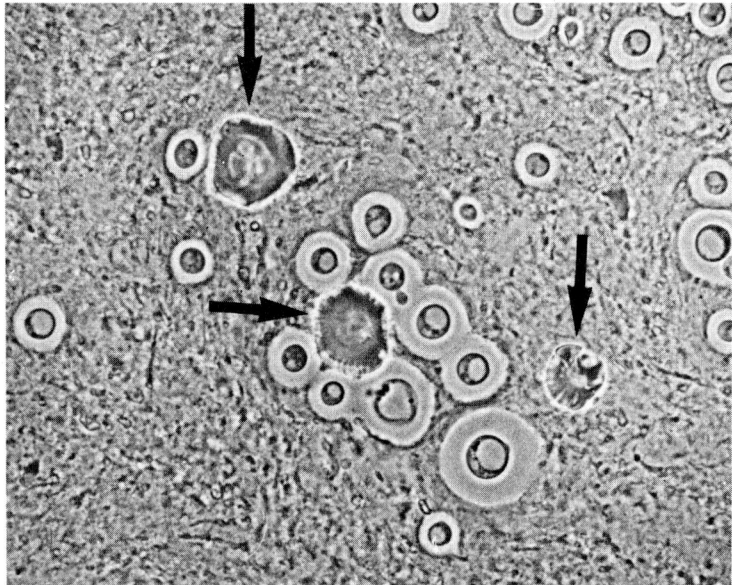

Fig. 4. Highly encapsulated budding cells and degenerated forms of cryptococci (marked by the arrows) in the squash preparation from the eye of the same mouse shown in Fig. 1. × 620

which was confirmed by histopathological and microbiological examinations. Interestingly, *C. neoformans* could be isolated only from the eyes of two of these mice – one control and one glycerine-treated animal. Thus strain W 2/A 94, besides causing selective involvement of the brain, can also cause selective involvement of the eye. It should be noted that involvement of the eye was significantly higher in the glycerine-treated mice (14%) than in the controls (2%). In the affected animals, the acute stage of the infection showed a tendency to heal spontaneously, leaving, however, permanent blindness. Surprisingly, this *C. neoformans* strain could be isolated from only 20% of the glycerine-administered mice, in contrast to 60% of the controls, when all surviving animals were killed at 8 weeks.

Fig. 2. Cryptococcoma shown in Fig. 1 at higher magnification, illustrating isolated chorioretinitis and several encapsulated cryptococci. PAS stain, × 560

Fig. 3. Another area from the lesion shown in Fig. 1, illustrating intraocular granulomatous tissue with relatively less dense cryptococci, mostly nonencapsulated and phagocytized. PAS stain, × 450

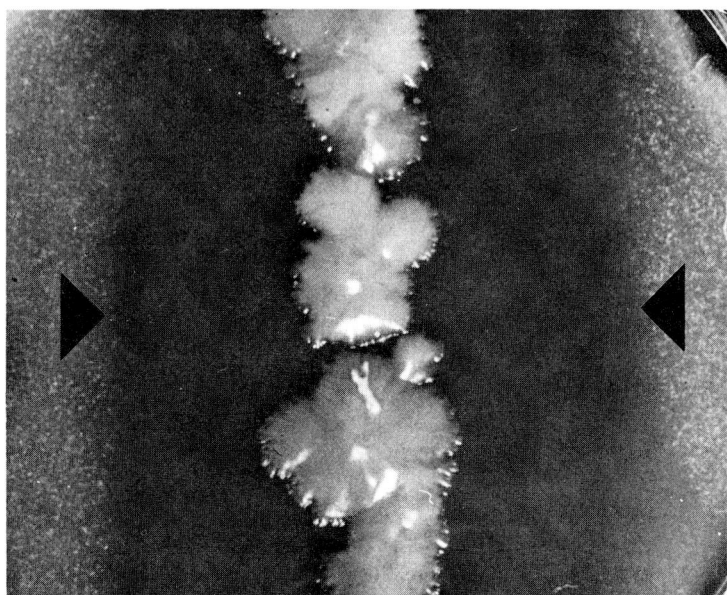

Fig. 5. Three weeks old mucoid growth of *C. neoformans* strain W 71/A 117 on uric acid agar, showing solubilization of uric acid crystals (indicated by the arrows).

Effect of Uric Acid on C. neoformans:

All the 31 strains of *C. neoformans* grew equally well on the media containing uric acid, urea or creatinine as sole source of nitrogen (*Staib et al.*, 1976c). In nine strains, the growth on uric acid agar (the basal medium containing uric acid as sole source of nitrogen) was accompanied by solubilization of uric acid crystals (Fig. 5); incidentally, six of these strains were highly virulent for white mice. However, colonies of 20 strains appeared more mucoid on uric acid agar as compared to their normal, mucoid appearance on other media, including SDA and *Guizotia* abyssinica-creatinine agar. Moreover, there was usually a distinct increase in capsule size which was more marked in those strains which had small to medium sized capsules. The 11 strains which formed dry-looking colonies on SDA and had no capsule initially, showed more or less similar characteristics on uric acid agar. However, after about one week, sectors of moderate to heavy mucoid growth appeared along with the primary dry growth in the case of eight strains. This growth remained mucoid when subcultured on SDA or uric acid agar, and was composed of spherical cells, surrounded by large capsules ranging from $2-4\,\mu$ in thickness. The 48 hour old subcultures from a mucoid colony of one of these strains (W 71/A 117) grown at 26°C on uric acid agar and SDA were tested for virulence in white mice. Groups of mice were inoculated

(2×10^7 cells/ml/mouse) i.p. as well as by the intramuscular route (4×10^6 cells/ml/mouse). The animals were observed over a period of 4 months. Contrary to the well known characteristics of the original strain W 71/A 117 (*Staib et al.,* 1974; *Staib and Mishra* 1975a, b), none of the i.m. inoculated mice showed any evidence of "cryptococcoma" formation at the site of inoculation and the over-all mortality was strikingly low and delayed.

Discussion

These observations demonstrate that there are *C. neoformans* strains which can survive solely in the brain of white mice for three months (or longer) following i.p. inoculation. They cause destruction of the brain by formation of solitary or multiple "cryptococcoma", in about 5% of the animals. These findings lead us to the conclusion that *C. neoformans* possesses strain-specific properties in relation to virulence for white mice, and organ-specificity. In humans, usually selective involvement of the brain is observed, unlike the general involvement of numerous organs mostly reported in experimental cryptococcosis in mice. However, as was shown with the *C. neoformans* strain W 2/A 94 and five others described here, there do exist strains which behave during the course of experimental infection in white mice as *C. neoformans* usually does in man as the aetiologic agent of cryptococcosis. Since with strain W 2/A 94 not only selective involvement of the brain could be caused in the mice, but also involvement of the eye (or both together), it appears that the eye, under certain circumstances, behaves more or less as a part of the CNS as far as the pathogenesis of cryptococcosis is concerned. In this context, the significance of "cryptococcoma" formation should be borne in mind. The "cryptococcoma", whether caused in an infected muscle by a general mouse-virulent strain (*Staib,* 1962a; *Staib et al.,* 1974; *Grosse et al.,* 1975b) or in the brain or eye by a so-called "mouse-avirulent, but brain-specific strain" must be accepted as the pathological-anatomical criterion of cryptococcosis. The "cryptococcoma" is characterized by a heavy growth of *C. neoformans* in a limited space and by absence of tissue reaction; it has *per se* certain pathological implications, depending on its location. Its progress demands growth of the connective tissue of the organ in which it is located, which is possible only by sufficient vascularisation (Fig. 6). Therefore, vascularisation has to be considered as a nutritional condition for *C. neoformans* growth. Furthermore, the vascularisation of "cryptococcoma" is of interest in connection with the large amounts of antigen in the blood during progressive cryptococcosis. From the therapy viewpoint also, the vascularisation of "cryptococcoma" is of significance as was shown in the animal experiments of *Grosse et al* (1975b). They clearly demonstrated the antimycotic action of amphotericin B around the blood capillaries in the "crytococcoma".

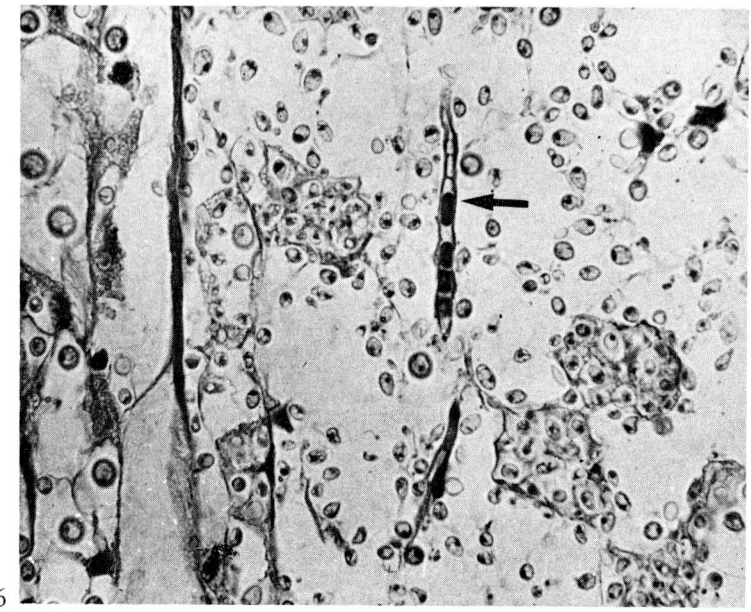

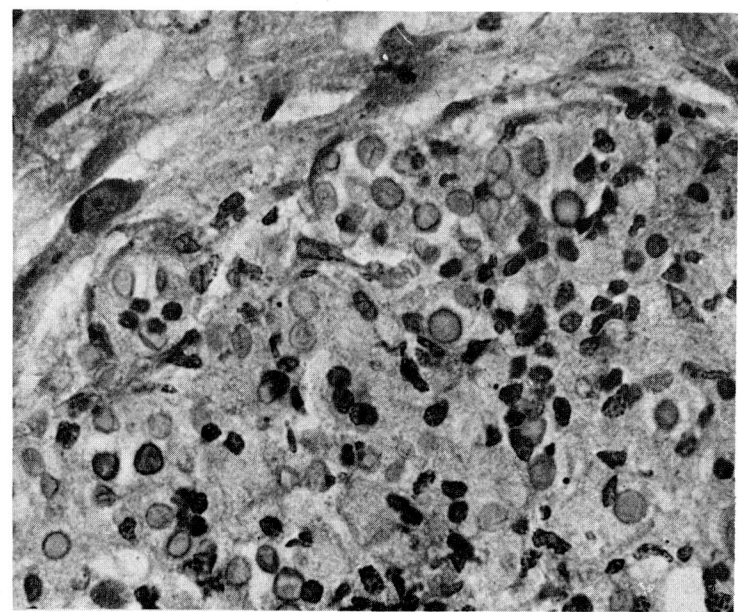

Special attention should be paid to a tendency for spontaneous healing of "cryptococcoma" (Fig. 7) in experimental animals (*Grosse et al.*, 1975a) and in man.

In experimental and clinical studies (*Staib et al.*, 1976a) we were able to show that a "cryptococcoma" can develop solely in the eye and heal spontaneously — leaving behind however possible loss of vision. Since the spontaneous healing of "cryptococcoma" is combined with a subsequent inflammatory process, mostly in the late stage of infection, the grossly manifest symptoms which start to develop are observed late in the course of the disease. Therefore, because of the inability to detect the fungus at this stage, difficulties in diagnosis are encountered.

We have observed cryptococcosis of the eye in a patient (*Erhorn et al.*, 1976) in whom uremia was the only underlying disease and the inflammatory granulomatous process in the eye began when the uremia was controlled. This poses a question regarding the influence of the uremia. Was it of nutritive significance, for instance with regard to organ-specific accumulation of low molecular weight nitrogenous substances, or did it influence the immunological reactions in the involved organ? Our observations on the involvement of the eye in mice in which uremia was induced artificially provide some relevant information. Our findings on the strain of *C. neoformans* (W 71/A 117) known to be highly virulent for white mice, are also of interest in this context. This strain produced no capsules on SDA and grew as dry colonies. However, when uric acid was provided as the sole source of nitrogen, morphological changes occurred which were accompanied by a distinct loss of virulence for white mice. Hence it appears that the virulence of the fungus may be affected by the low molecular weight nitrogenous-substances which are available (*Staib*, 1962b, 1963c) in nature or in the target organism. Capsule formation in this respect is of interest; it has been a central question since the detection of cryptococcosis, to date.

In view of the fact that we have succeeded (*Staib and Mishra*, 1975a) in immunising mice, using a so-called "low-virulent strain" against infection by a "highly-virulent strain", the significance of immunity in the pathogenesis of cryptococcosis has to be kept in mind in addition to nutritional factors. Further studies are needed to show to what extent spontaneous healing, immunological

---

Fig. 6. Section through a "cryptococcoma" in the hind leg of a mouse that died 3 weeks after i.m. inoculation with *C. neoformans* strain W 71/A 117, showing encapsulated cryptococci, intact capillary containing erythrocytes (shown by the arrow) and phagocytosis of mostly nonencapsulated cells. Masson-Goldner stain, × 560

Fig. 7. Section through the brain of a mouse with selective involvement of the brain, killed 4 weeks after i.p. inoculation with *C. neoformans* strain W 2/A 94. Note a spontaneously healing intracerebral lesion with distinct glia reaction and loss of stainability of the nonencapsulated cryptococci. Klüver-Barrera stain, × 560 oil

factors and the influence of other basic diseases have to be considered, besides the antimycotic drugs, in the therapy of cryptococcosis. We believe that comparative studies on human cryptococcosis should be done in white mice, using certain representative strains. Special attention should be paid to "cryptococcoma" formation, particularly during studies on pathogenesis, therapy and serodiagnosis of cryptococcosis.

Summary

In continuation of our previous research, we have confirmed that there are strains of *Cryptococcus neoformans* which can survive only in the brain and eye of white mice. Such strains are proposed for comparative studies in experimental cryptococcosis. New aspects in the study of the pathogenesis of cryptococcosis are provided by the observation that ocular cryptococcosis was more commonly observed in uremic mice than in normal animals. The "cryptococcoma" and its vascularisation are discussed in relation to different aspects of the pathogenesis, diagnosis and therapy of cryptococcosis.

Acknowledgement

We are grateful to Miss A. Blisse, Miss A. Passow and Mr. W. Altmann for their technical assistance.

References

Erhorn, J.; Grosse, G.; Staib, F., and Wollensak, J.: Klinische Monatsblätter für Augenheilkunde, in press (1976).
Grosse, G.; Mishra, S.K., and Staib, F.: Selective involvement of the brain in experimental murine cryptococcosis II. Histopathological observations. Zbl. Bakt. Hyg. I. Abt. Orig. A. *233:* 106–122 (1975a).
Grosse, G.; Staib, F.; Radlmeier, E, and Preuss, W.: Cryptococcom und Amphotericin B. Tierexperimentelle Untersuchungen zur Therapie der Cryptococcose. 2. Mitteilung Patho-histologische Befunde. Zbl. Bakt. Hyg. I. Abt. Orig. A *230:* 518–533 (1975b).
Staib, F.: Cryptococcus neoformans in muscle tissue. Zbl. Bakt., I. Abt. Orig. *185:* 135–144 (1962a).
Staib, F.: Vogelkot, ein Nährsubstrat für die Gattung *Cryptococcus.* Zbl. Bakt., I. Abt. Orig. *186:* 233–247 (1962b).
Staib, F.: Bedeutung von Thiamin (Vitamin B1) für die Assimilierbarkeit von Kreatinin durch *Cryptococcus neoformans.* Zbl. Bakt., I. Abt. Orig. *190:* 115–131 (1963a).
Staib, F.: Zur Kreatinin-Kreatin-Assimilation in der Hefepilzdiagnostik. Zbl. Bakt., I. Abt. Orig. *191:* 429–432 (1963b).
Staib, F.,: New concepts in the occurrence and identification of *Cryptococcus neoformans.* Mycopathol (Den Haag) *19:* 143–145 (1963c).

Staib, F.: Das Serum-Reststickstoff-Auxanogramm (mit Spross – und Schimmelpilzen). Zbl. Bakt., I. Abt. Orig. *194:* 379–406 (1964).
Staib, F.; Preuss, W., and Radlmeier, E.: Cryptococcom und Amphoterich B. Tierexperimentelle Untersuchungen zur Therapie der cryptococcose. I. Mikrobiologische Befunde. Zbl. Bakt. Hyg., I. Abt. Orig. A *226:* 561–566 (1974).
Staib, F. and Mishra, S.K.: Contribution to the strain-specific virulence of *Cryptococcus neoformans.* Animal experiments with two *C. neoformans* strains isolated from bird manure. Zbl. Bakt. Hyg., 1, Abt. Orig. A *230:* 81–85 (1975a).
Staib, F. and Mishra, S.K.: Selective involvement of the brain in experimental murine cryptococcosis I. Microbiological observations. Zbl. Bakt. Hyg., I. Abt. Orig. A *232:* 355–364 (1975b).
Staib, F.; Mishra, S.K.; and Grosse, G.: VIth Congress International Soc. Human and Animal Mycology Tokyo/Japan, in press (1975).
Staib, F.; Mishra, S.K.; Grosse, G., and Abel, T.: Zbl. Bakt. Hyg. I., Abt. Orig., in press (1976a).
Staib, F.; Mishra, S.K.; Abel, T., and Blisse, A.: Zbl. Bakt. Hyg., I. Abt. Orig., in press (1976b).
Staib, F.; Mishra, S.K.; Abel, T., and Blisse, A.: Zbl. Bakt. Hyg., I. Abt. Orig., in press (1976c).
Thiel, G.; Wilson, D.T.; Arce, M.L., and Oken, D.E.: Glycerol induced hemoglobinuric acute renal failure in the rat. II. The experimental model, predisposing factors and pathophysiological features. Nephron *4:* 276–297 (1967).

Prof. Dr. Dr. *F. Staib,* Robert Koch Institut, Nordufer 20 *D–100 Berlin 65* (FRG)

Cinematography and Scanning Electron Microscopy of Leukocytic Rings Formed *in vitro* Around *Cryptococcus neoformans*

A. Shahar, Yehudith Kletter and M. Aronson

Israel Institute for Biological Research, Ness Ziona and Sackler School of Medicine, Tel-Aviv University, Tel-Aviv

Introduction

Cryptococcus neoformans was used as a model to investigate cellular reactions to large-sized parasites. In our previous studies on cellular reactions to yeast using light and transmission electron microscopy, we found that phagocytic cells which cannot phagocytize the yeast due to its large dimensions (50–70 μm) surround it and form ring-like structures (*Schneerson-Porat et al.*, 1965; *Shahar*, 1968). The ring formations lead to the destruction of the yeast by the phagocytic cells through a mechanism in which humoral and cellular factors are involved (*Shahar et al.*, 1969; *Aronson and Kletter*, 1973; *Kalina et al.*, 1974).

To obtain a better understanding, we have further studied the ring structures using time-lapse cinematography and scanning electron microscopy (SEM). The process of ring formation and the surface structure of the yeast and of the phagocytic cells are described here.

Materials and Methods

C. neoformans was grown on the medium devised by *Littman and Tsubura* (1959) for obtaining large capsulated yeasts. Preparations were routinely counted and checked by India-ink smears to ascertain cell size. For observation, the 48-hour cultures were centrifuged and resuspended in Tyrode's solution.

Cultures of phagocytic cells. Polymorphonuclears and macrophages were harvested from the peritoneal cavity of rabbits 18 or 120 hours respectively after injection with 0.2% starch solution. For SEM, 10^6 phagocytic cells and 10^4 large-sized cryptococci were cultured in a medium consisting of 40% rabbit serum in Tyrode's solution, in Leighton tubes; the tubes were incubated at 37° for 5 hours. For cinematography, leukocytes were mixed with cryptococci and were allowed to settle on a cover-glass at 37°. The cover-glass was subsequently mounted in a paraffin oil-filled chamber and sealed with paraffin (fig. 1).

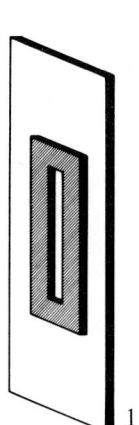 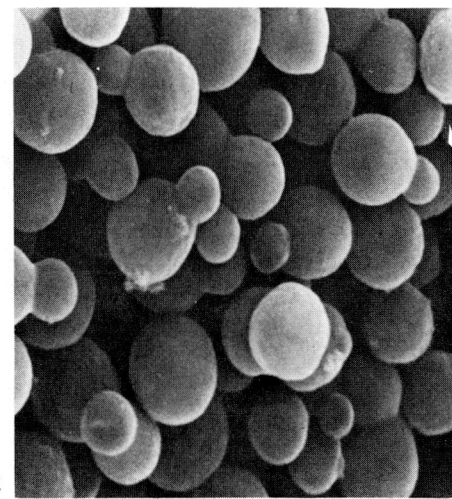

Fig. 1. Observation chamber for cinematography (× 1.1). The shaded portion is made of stainless steel, and is glued onto a glass slide.

Fig. 2. A group of 'naked' cryptococci which have lost their capsules after 30 minutes' incubation in glutaraldehyde and acetone. SEM. × 6000.

Time-lapse cinematography was then employed at a speed of 15 frames per minute, using a phase contrast microscope (Zeiss microcine camera).

Scanning electron microscopy. The yeast cells were prepared either as pellets, or attached to cover glasses previously coated with a polaroid fixative. Preparations were fixed in 2% glutaraldehyde for 10–30 minutes. Dehydration was accomplished in increments of ethanol and acetone.

The preparations on cover slips were critical-point dried in a Polaron C.P.D. apparatus using liquid CO_2 and the pellet preparations by the method of *Jones and Gillett* (1975).

Cover glasses with cultured phagocytic cells and yeasts were fixed in 2% glutaraldehyde for 30 minutes, dehydrated as above and critical-point dried.

SEM was carried out using an ISI superminiscan II at 15 KV on specimens vacuum-coated with 250–350 Å gold (Polaron spattering unit).

Results and Discussion

Morphological Appearance of C. neoformans *as Visualized by SEM*

Electron microscopy of fungal cells is notoriously difficult. Artifacts are commonly found as result of conventional fixation and embedding procedures (*Edwards et al.,* 1967). We therefore modified the fixation technique by 1) shortening the glutaraldehyde fixation time to 10 min; 2) shortening the acetone dehydration time to 5 min; 3) employing critical point drying. These modifications yielded optimal conditions for capsule preservation (fig. 2, 3). The crypto-

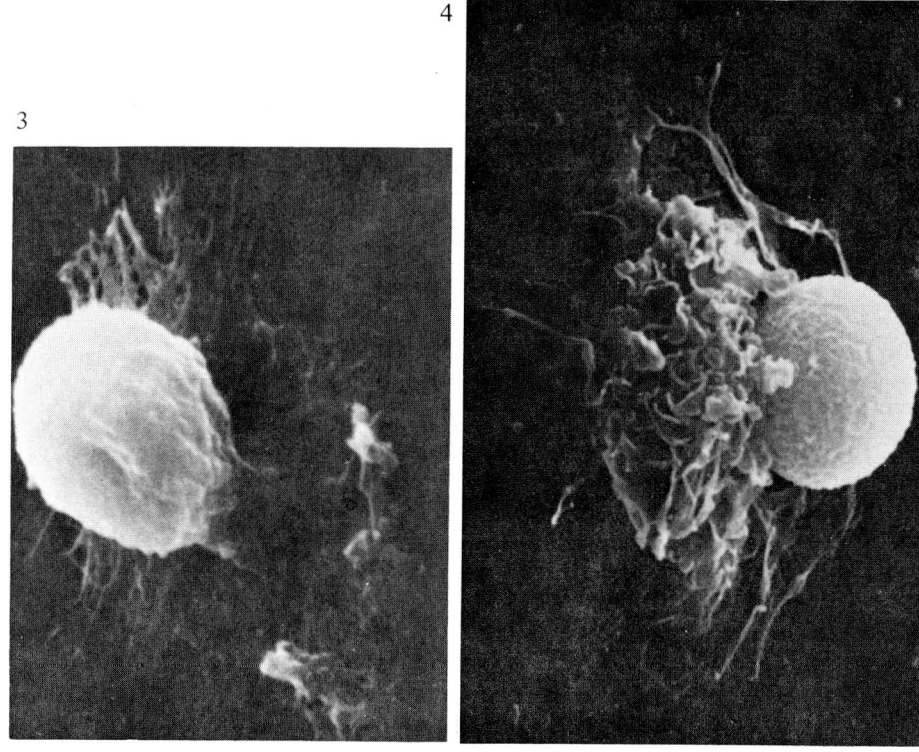

Fig. 3. A well-encapsulated yeast (from the same culture as in Fig. 2). Fixation and dehydration in acetone were shortened to 10 min and 5 min respectively. SEM. × 4500.
Fig. 4. A macrophage attempting to phagocytize a cryptococcus. SEM. × 4500.

coccus resembles a miniature golf-ball covered with appendages which are presumably the capsule filaments described by *Edwards et al.* (1967).

Better preservation of the capsule was obtained in the samples of yeast cells which adhered to cover glasses than in those prepared as pellets.

Morphology of the Ring Structure

The first stage toward formation of rings is the adherence of a pseudopodium of a phagocytic cell (polymorphonuclear or macrophage) to the yeast cell, presumably in a futile attempt to phagocytose it. This was seen both by cinematography and SEM (fig. 4).

Later, additional cells encircle the *Cryptococcus,* but only restricted areas of the yeast are seen to be attached by the pseudopodia of the macrophages, which remain apart from one another (fig. 5, 6).

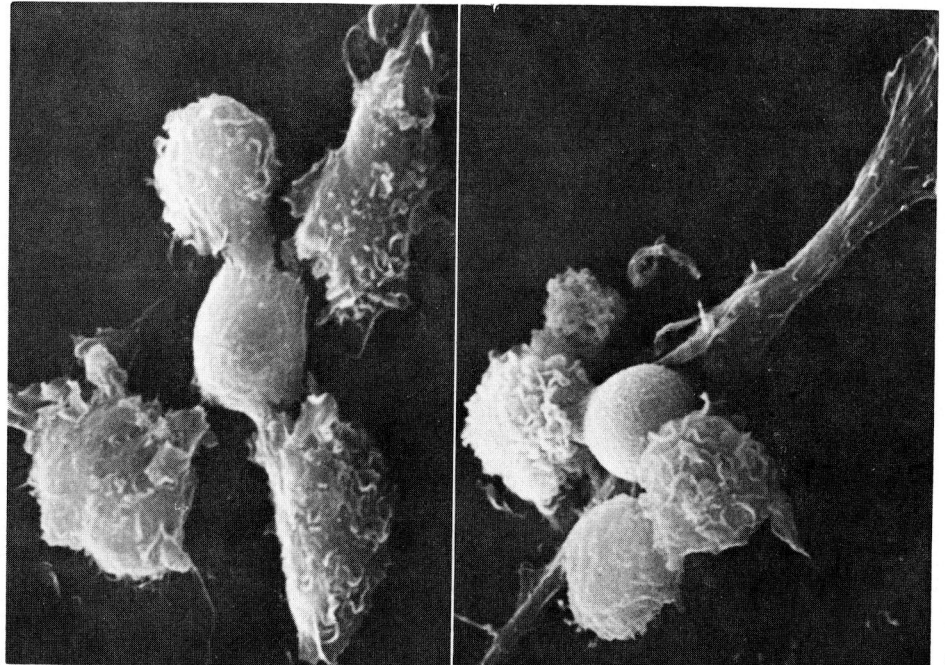

Fig. 5, 6. Macrophages in the process of forming a ring around *Cryptococcus neoformans* 5 hours after onset of culture. SEM. × 2700.

In the "mature" ring, many of the pseudopodia of the phagocytic cells are attached to the part of the *Cryptococcus* which is in contact with the cover glass, and no distinction can be made between them and the yeast capsule. At this stage, firm connections are also formed among the cells composing the ring, presumably lending stability to the ring structure (fig. 7). However, the ring is always two-dimensional, leaving the upper part of the *Cryptococcus* uncovered by the phagocytic cells.

One of the peculiar aspects of the ring reaction is that the phagocytic cells surround the *Cryptococcus* at its sides but do not encapsulate it; i.e., the response is 2-dimensional and not 3-dimensional. The possible reasons for this phenomenon have been discussed (*Shahar et al.,* 1969), and it has also been shown that in the presence of large quantities of immune serum, 3-dimensional structures are obtained (*Aronson and Kletter,* 1973). It was nevertheless desirable to ascertain that under normal *in vitro* conditions the rings are indeed 2-dimensional and that this apparent feature is not the result of an optical illusion; the use of SEM and cinematography served as a convenient way to establish the steric structure of the ring.

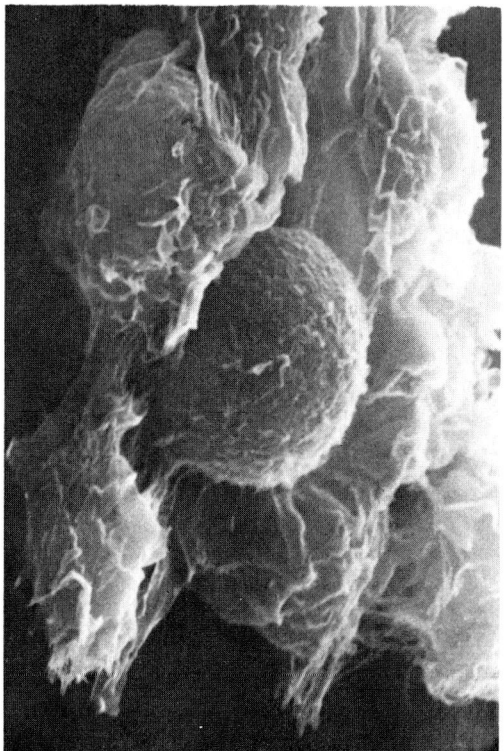

Fig. 7. A complete ("mature") ring. SEM. × 4500.

Acknowledgements

The authors wish to thank Mrs. *Rina Mordechai* for her valuable technical assistance and Mr. *P. Hadas* for the photographic prints.

References

Aronson, M. and Kletter, Y.: Aspects of the defense against a large-sized parasite, the yeast, *Cryptococcus neoformans;* in *Zuckerman and Weiss* Dynamic aspects of host-parasite relationships, vol 1, pp. 132–162 (1973).
Edwards, M.R.; Gordon, M.A.; Laja, E.W., and Ghiorse, W.C.: Micromorphology of *Cryptococcus neoformans.* J. Bact. *94:* 766–777 (1967).
Jones, G.E. and Gillett, R.: A simple method of preparing a cell suspension for scanning electron microscopy. Experientia *31:* 1244 (1975).

Kalina, M.; Kletter, Y., and Aronson, M.: The interaction of phagocytes and the large sized parasite *Cryptococcus neoformans:* cytochemical and ultrastructural study. Cell Tiss. Res. *152:* 165–174 (1974).

Littman, M.H. and Tsubura, E.: Effect of degree of encapsulation upon virulence of *Cryptococcus neoformans.* Proc. Soc. exp. Biol. Med. *101:* 773–777 (1959).

Shahar, A.: Some aspects of the defense mechanism against *Cryptococcus neoformans.* Proc. Acad. Med. Torino *131:* 7–12, 140 (1968).

Shahar, A.; Kletter, Y., and Aronson, M.: Granuloma formation in cryptococcosis. Israel J. med. Scis. *5/6:* 1164–1172 (1969).

Schneerson-Porat, S.; Shahar, A., and Aronson, M.: Formation of histocyte rings in response to *Cryptococcus neoformans* infection. J. reticuloendoth. Soc. *2:* 249–255 (1965).

Dr. *A. Shahar,* Israel Institute for Biological Research, *Ness Ziona* (Israel)

Discussion

Dr. *Louria:* Is the situation similar with human leukocytes? How do your studies relate to those of *Diamond* and colleagues showing phagocytosis by human polymorphonuclear leukocytes?

Dr. *Shahar:* The situation is similar in cultures of human leukocytes. Phagocytosis and ring formation are obtained in these cultures, but mostly by macrophages.

Pathogenesis of Mucocutaneous Mycoses Caused by Yeasts

O. Male

1st Dermatological University Clinic, Medical School, Vienna, Austria

Introduction

Banal mycoses of the skin and the adjacent mucous membranes caused by *Candida* species and related yeasts have become increasingly more widespread, and constitute today one of the most frequently occurring dermatological infectious diseases. At the same time, there is a new tendency for spread of such infections even to inner organs and/or to septicemia, opportunistic infections which virtually constitute new diseases. Detailed knowledge of the changing aspects of *Candida* infections forms the basis of successful prophylaxis and therapy, and since the principles of definition and nomenclature of fungi have changed considerably in recent years and are quite unfamiliar to non-mycologists, they will now be summarised.

Definition and Nomenclature

From the etiological viewpoint, only those mycoses are candidoses (CA) that are caused by *Candida* (*C.*) species. There is, however, another group of mycoses, clinically and histologically identical with the "true" candidoses, which are caused by species of other *cryptococcacea* genera closely related to *Candida*. These are primarily *Torulopsis* species and more rarely *Trigonopsis, Kloeckera, Brettanomyces, Trichosporon* species and others. The causal agent in these infections is *C. albicans* in 85–90 per cent of cases and *C. parapsilosis, C. tropicalis, C. stellatoidea, C. krusei, C. guilliermondii* in 3–5 per cent of cases of true candidoses. *Torulopsis* (*T.*) *glabrata, T. albicans, T. minor* and *T. inconspicua* account for 5–8 per cent of cases of the candidoses-like mycoses and about 2 per cent are due to other species (*Louria et al.*, 1967; *Gonzales-Mendoza* and *Aguirre-Garcia*, 1967; *Male*, 1971; *Drouhet*, 1972; *Scholer*, 1974a).

Diagnosis of such cases, above all the distinction of CA-like mycoses from true candidosis can be effected only by complicated procedures for identification of the fungi in question. As the appropriate facilities for such tests are not always available, most practising physicians usually consider all clinically CA-like mycoses as candidosis when their causative yeasts do not differ in their cultural behavior from *Candida* species. In practice, this is acceptable because the CA-like mycoses usually behave like the "true" CA from the therapeutic viewpoint. However, for the sake of correct definition, lately, the following provisional regulation has been proposed: the term *"levurosis"* represents all mycoses caused by *C.*-species and *C.*-like banal yeasts; the former are named "true" CA, the latter "CA-like" mycoses. The nosological counterpart to the levuroses are the "classical yeast mycoses" like cryptococcosis, histoplasmosis, coccidioidomycosis, sporotrichosis, blastomycosis, etc. Only "true" CA will be discussed here.

Epidemiology

The origin and mode of infection by *Candida* do not require much discussion. The fungi are so common and so widely distributed in the environment — for example — in water (especially bathing water), on fruits, vegetables and milk products, and, indeed, on human beings themselves, especially as saprophytes in the digestive tract (*Male*, 1964; *Rieth and Wildfeuer*, 1976), that there is practically current, if not permanent, exposure (*Winner and Hurley*, 1964; *Bernhardt*, 1968, 1973; *Huhn*, 1971; *Scholer*, 1974b). Quantitatively, however, they are generally insufficient to cause infection under physiological conditions.

Pathogenesis

A most important and currently much discussed question is whether the CA represent a primary or a secondary disease and whether its organisms are pathogenic or opportunistic (*Louria et al.*, 1960, 1967; *Male*, 1964, 1971, 1973a, b; *Kozinn and Taschdjian*, 1966; *Lehner and Ward*, 1970; *Marget and Schwab*, 1971; *Scholer*, 1974b; *Auger and Joly*, 1975). The reason why these questions are so important is that the process in the first case depends mainly on the pathogenic properties of the organisms, while in the latter, the condition of the host is of predominant importance. These considerations affect the infection itself, the type of mycosis, the character of the lesions, the course and prognosis of the disease, as well as how and where treatment should be directed — to the parasite only in the primary process, or, in the secondary process, aimed at the elimination or normalization of the predisposing factors in the host.

HOST-PARASITE-RELATIONSHIPS
❶ NONPATHOGENIC ❷ PATHOGENIC ❸ OPPORTUNISTIC

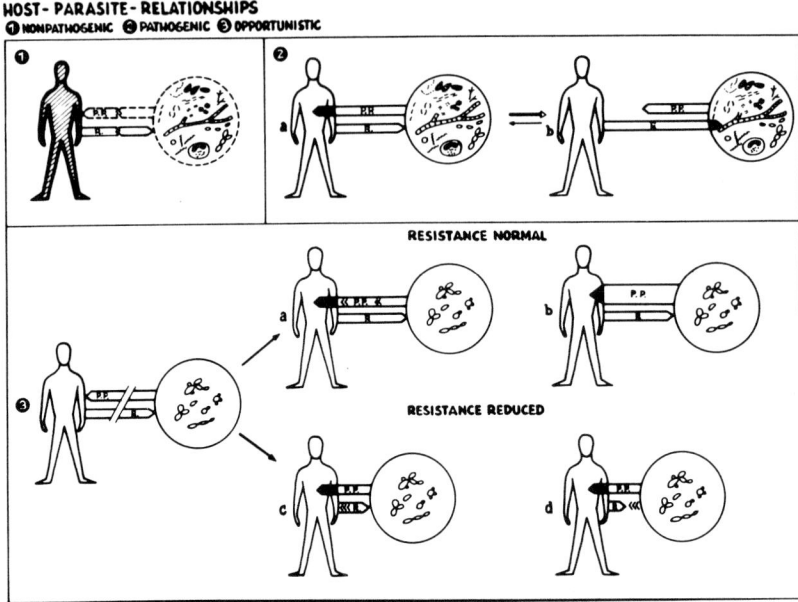

Fig. 1. Pathogenetic host-parasite relationships in 1) nonpathogenic, 2) pathogenic and 3) opportunistic yeasts. Explanation is given in the text.

We know today that the CA may be primary or secondary, but that the proportion of primary and secondary pathogenicity is not a fixed one, changing with the prevailing ecological and medical conditions and level of civilisation. Secondly, boundaries between primary and secondary CA are sometimes quite indistinct and subject to subjective opinion. The secondary CA are today by far the most frequent, and at the same time medically the most important. As such superimposed diseases are determined first of all by their pathogenesis, the latter will now be discussed in more detail.

In principle, the pathogenesis of an infectious disease is determined by two components: by the pathogenic properties of the causative germs and by the host defensive mechanisms. Let us conceive theoretically possible constellations in the host-parasite relationships, as represented schematically in Fig. 1. Though this representation is rather elementary, it is useful because the situation concerning the opportunistic yeasts does not entirely correspond with conventional ideas.

With respect to their pathogenicity, yeasts are divided into *non-pathogenic*, *pathogenic* and *facultatively pathogenic* classes. (The same is true more or less for all other organisms but here only the yeasts are discussed).

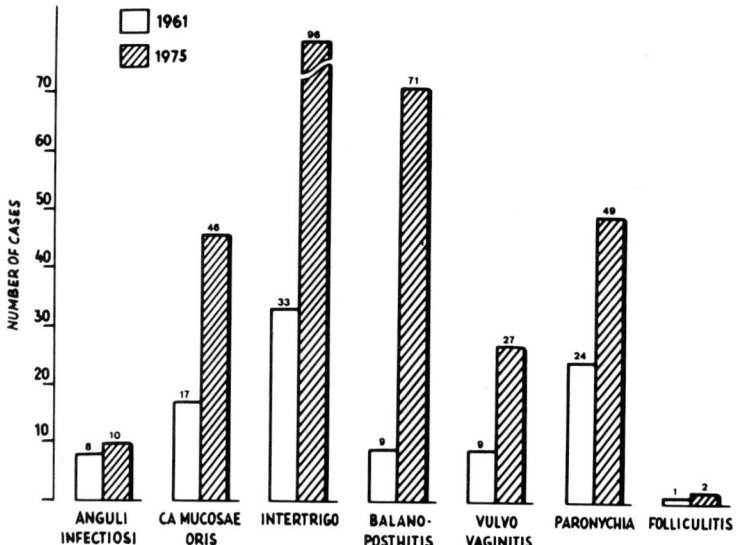

Fig. 2. Spectrum and frequency of mucocutaneous candidoses observed in the 1st Dermatological Clinic, University of Vienna, in 1961 and 1975.

A yeast is *non-pathogenic* only if the host conditions are absolutely incompatible with its metabolism, i.e. if it is not able to metabolize the building materials or the excretion products of the host, or becomes inactivated by them, or cannot tolerate its environment [Fig. 1 (1)].

A yeast is *pathogenic* if its pathogenic potencies (pp) are more powerful than the defence factors of the non-immunised host under physiological conditions. In the case of immunisation, the resistance of the host may become the prevailing factor [Fig. 1 (2)].

A yeast is *facultatively pathogenic* if its pp are weaker than the resistance of the host only to the extent that under normal conditions the host resistance prevails but, under abnormal conditions, the pp may overcome host resistance. It is generally assumed that a facultatively pathogenic yeast can only become pathogenic if the host resistance is lowered by endogenous or exogenous factors [Fig. 1 (3c and d)], but this is not always true. Such yeasts can become parasitic in a relatively high percentage of cases also when the resistance of the host is normal. Under these circumstances, there are two possibilities: either the pp of the yeast increase *qualitatively* [Fig. 1 (3a)] or the number of yeasts increases *quantitatively* [Fig. 1 (3b)] to such a degree that the defence of the host is overpowered.

The former, augmentation of virulence, can be induced, *e.g.* by steroids and certain sex hormones (*Catterali,* 1966; *Daniel,* 1972). Massive multiplication of

Table I. Predisposing factors for infections caused by opportunistic yeasts

I. *Exogenous*

1) *Influence of the environment*
   a) physical
      maceration, angiospasms
   b) chemical
      solvents, detergents, cleaning and/or bleaching agents, disinfectants, etc.
2) *Interaction between the organisms and chemicals or mechanical irritation*
   a) pharmaceutical products, e.g. steroids
   b) mechanical agents, e.g., catheters, valves, prostheses
3) *Influence of precedent or simultaneous infections*
   T. rubrum, Staphylococcus aureus, B. pyocyaneum, Trichomonas vaginalis

II. *Indirectly endogenous*

1) *Ecologically effective*
   antibiotics (tetracyclines, aminoglycosides)
2) *Lowering the resistance*
   steroids, immunosuppressives, cytostatics, actinic effects, heroin
3) *Others*
   sex hormones, especially gestagens

III. *Endogenous*

1) *Anomalies of circulation*
   a) concerning only single parts of the vessels
      mostly arterial, rarely venous
   b) concerning the entire circulation
      mostly congenital cardiac defects
2) *Systemic diseases*
   malignancies, hepato- and nephro-pathies
3) *Endocrinopathies*
   diabetes (essential and steroid-induced), *Cushing*'s disease, hypothyroidism
4) *Immunopathies with congenital defects*
   progressive septic granulomatosis, myeloperoxydase deficiency, hereditary displasia of thymus (*Nezelof-Allibone*),
   Di George's syndrome, *Chediak Higashi Steinbrinck*'s syndrome,
   Swiss type of agammaglobulinemia.

yeasts — which incidentally is of specific medical significance — is caused primarily by antibiotics. Sometimes the increase of the pp of the yeast and the lowering of the host's resistance occur simultaneously.

By far the most important part in the facultative pathogenicity is played by those factors which cause a lowering of the resistance of the host. Those which are known to us are listed in Table I. They may be either 1) *exogenic,* 2) *indirectly endogenic* and 3) *endogenic* and/or constitutional, conditional or accidental. Of course, mixed as well as transitional forms are possible. The exogenic factors cause practically only localized CA involving the skin and the adjacent mucous membranes. The direct and indirect endogenic factors cause almost exclusively systematic infections. The pathomechanisms of particular disposing factors can be understood from the description of the clinical forms of CA which they cause (Fig. 2). The most affected tissues are the skin (epidermis) and/or mucous membrane, the nail and the hair; sometimes the conditions in the patient are not clearly confined. Our data are taken from the cases seen during the last 15 years at the 1st Dermatological University Clinic in Vienna (Fig. 2).

Clinical forms of CA

A) Forms affecting mainly the epidermis and/or the mucous membranes

1) *CA of the angles of the mouth without involvement of the oral mucosa (anguli infectiosi candidamycetici)*

Usually occurring in the elderly (average age 52 years), about 95 per cent have dentures. The sex incidence, m:f, is 2:3. Pathogenesis: badly fitting prosthesis; apposition of upper and lower lip; wrinkling at the angles of the mouth; maceration of the epithelium (possibly caused by incompatibility of the prosthetic material and/or disinfectants); nosoparasitic involvement by saprophytes of the oral mucosa; or contamination by food.

2) *CA of the oral mucosa (CA* mucosae oris*) with or without involvement of the angles of the mouth*

a) *Chronic form, prognostically unfavorable.* Mostly occurring in older patients (average age 55 years) with a long-lasting, eventually incurable, general disease, or pathologic disorders of the entire organism (i.e. hemoblastoses, reticuloses, malignant processes, autoimmune aggressions, other immunopathies, immune defects and endocrinopathies (*Mirsky and Cuttner,* 1960; *Dourov and Doustin,* 1964; *Dennis et al.,* 1968; *Lehrer and Cline,* 1969; *Montes et al.,* 1972; *Kecht,* 1973; *Chen and Webster,* 1974).

b) *Acute form, prognostically more favorable.* Usually occurring in younger adults (average age 23 years) accompanied by a transitory lowering of the general state of well-being, mainly after severe accidents, shock, infectious diseases, etc. Found especially in intensive care wards (*Dennis et al.,* 1968; *Law et al.,* 1972; *MacMillan et al.,* 1972; *Vust and Grigoriu,* 1973; *Kecht,* 1973; *Rayner,* 1973).

Both infections originate usually from the oral mucosa saprophytes. More rarely, they are "hospitalism" germs. They become pathogenic because of a defect in the host defence caused by therapy (immunosuppressives, cytostatics, steroids, etc.) and in b) usually due to the original disease or trauma. Both CA-forms are often aggravated by antibiotic therapy, indirectly by suppresssion of bacterial contaminants and directly by stimulation of growth of mycetes (*Lipnik et al.,* 1952; *Seelig,* 1966; *Chotiner and Piver,* 1971; *Curry and Quie,* 1971).

c) *CA* mucosae oris neonatorum. α) harmless form, occurring relatively frequently, in dyspepsia (especially in artificially nourished infants), healing usually spontaneously without therapeutic difficulties. β) grave form, occurring rarely, e.g. in congenital cardiac vitia or immune defects; often together with onychomycosis and granulomatous CA of the skin and/or scalp (*Higgs and Wells,* 1974; *Mobacken and Lindholm,* 1974; *Schirar et al.,* 1974).

The fungi originate mostly from the maternal birth canals. Sometimes they are "hospitalism" yeasts. In untreated and/or especially severe cases of a) and b) and c)-β, other mucous membranes and parts of the skin may become involved, resulting in, eventually, mycotic septicemia with widespread infection of many organs and death. However, the mycosis usually remains localized in the circumscribed areas. On the other hand, very often the number of saprophytic yeasts of the intestinal tract increases considerably, leading in some cases to dissemination of mycotic germs and absorption of toxins and allergens. They may also constitute at least a focus of infection. Furthermore, the proliferation of yeasts causes an alteration in the normal intestinal flora and therefore a disturbance of the balance of vitamins through biotin requirements. They may thus impair the normal courses of digestion and resorption (*Male,* 1967; *Seebacher,* 1972).

3) *CA of intertriginous areas (*intertrigo candidamycetica*)*

a) *Trunk (infra-mammary, inguinal region, anal cleft, abdominal folds).* Occurring in adults, mainly in cases of diabetes and adipositas, sometimes with disturbances listed under 2 a) and b), average age 44 years, sex incidence, m:f = 24:76.

Origin of yeast: mainly feces, and — in women — saprophytes of the vaginal mucosa (transferred to more distant body regions by towels and bathing water), and the maternal birth canals; sometimes "hospitalism" and "environmental" yeasts (*Lachenicht and Potel,* 1971). Exogenous infections caused by suction teats and pacifiers also lead to the colonization of the intestinal tract (*Blaschke-Hellmessen,* 1971). In the inguinocrural and perianal region, the CA are occasionally (3 per cent of cases) combined with a dermatophytosis caused almost

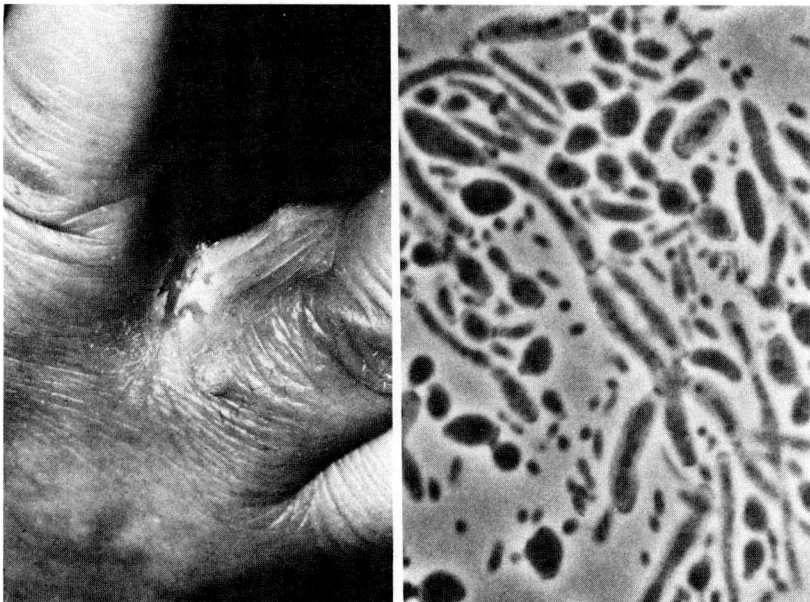

Fig. 3. Erosio interdigitalis mycetica found in a washerwoman; clinically in a KOH preparation indistinguishable from a candidosis. Causative yeast (on the right hand side) *Trichosporon cutaneum.* × 480.

always by *Trichophyton rubrum.* Pathogenesis: enhancement of mycotic infection due to the increased glycogen content; moisture and maceration of the epithelium. Precipitating factor: creation of a "moist chamber" by the now generally used diaper trousers.

b) *Interdigital spaces of the hands (*erosio candidamycetica interdigitalis manus*).* Occurring practically only in adults (average age 35 years), sex incidence, m:f = 24:76, mostly in persons who are continually in contact with — especially cold — water, (bio)detergents, etc. For example, washerwomen, housewives, bar personnel (Fig. 3). In 25 per cent of cases — generally the longer-lasting and severe ones — an additional CA-paronychia occurs.

Origin of the yeasts: diapers, other (soaking) laundry, dregs of beer ("wild yeasts"), environmental germs. Pathogenesis: disturbance of the cutaneous acid secretions and capacity for neutralization of alkali; maceration of the epithelium by chemicals and continual dampness.

c) *Interdigital spaces of the feet (*erosio candidamycetica interdigitalis pedis*).* This is the most rare form of epidermal CA, occurring only in adults (average age 39 years), usually in men (sex incidence, m:f = 81:19), especially in

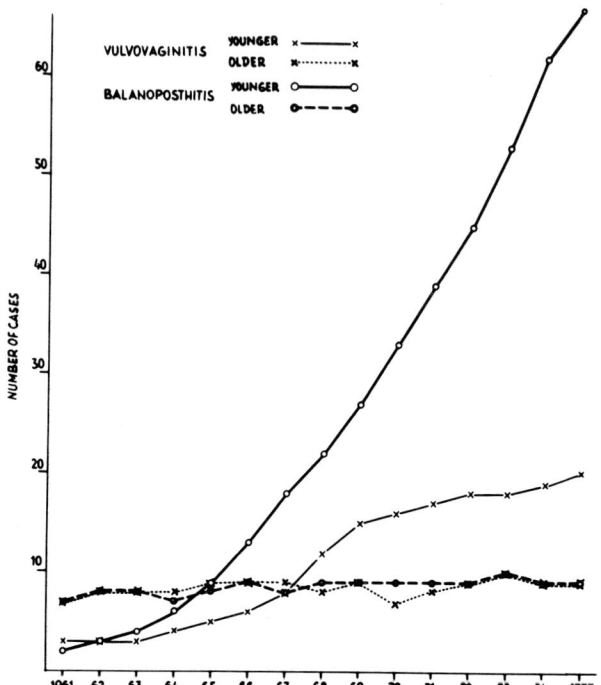

Fig. 4. Frequency of vulvovaginitis and balanoposthitis caused by *Candida spp.* observed in our clinic from 1961 to 1976.

persons who are continuously in a damp and warm environment and wear airtight footwear like rubber or plastic boots (miners, cellar and laundry workers; colour-spray-lacquerers, *etc.*). In about 12 per cent of cases, dermatophytosis is also present. In addition, there is often a remarkable abundance of (nosoparasitic) bacteria, mostly staphylococci and streptococci.

Predisposing factors: congestion due to heat and humidity; venous stasis and ischemia due to compression of the toes by footwear; and, in some cases, diabetes.

4) *CA of the genitals*

a) *Balanoposthitis candidamycetica.* The state was relatively rarely diagnosed until 10 years ago and occurred almost only in older patients with diabetes and/or kraurosis; nowadays it is seen more often in younger persons (Fig. 4). The average age in 82 per cent of our cases was 20 years; in 80 percent of these patients, the female partner took ovulation inhibitors, and in 14 per cent, the patients were pregnant. The remaining 18 per cent of patients had an

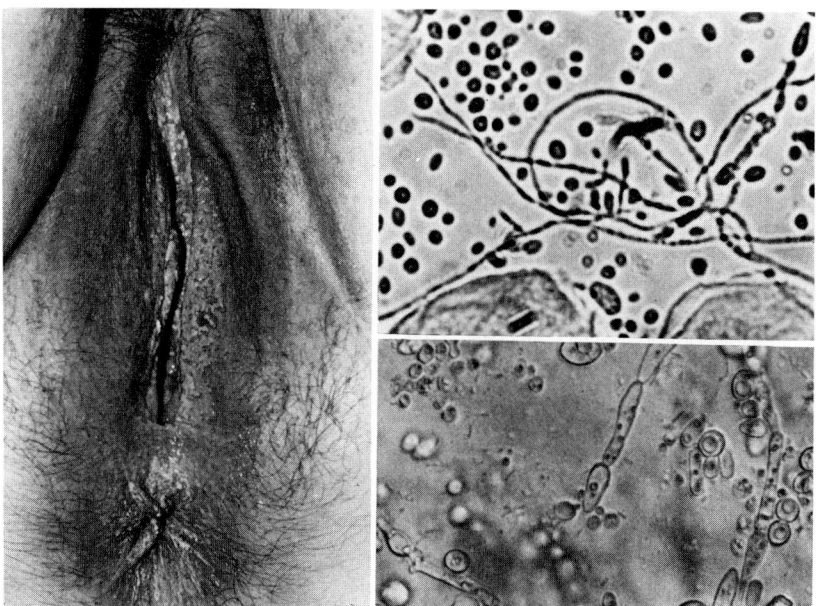

Fig. 5. Candidosis of genitals and anus in a severely burned patient. Direct examination of the gastric juice (top, right) and feces (bottom, right) after treatment of the patient with high doses of antibiotics for 4 weeks.

average age of 58 years, 95 per cent of them had diabetes, 3 per cent kraurosis.

Origin of yeast: female genitals, passage from other body regions. Predisposing factors: "moist chambers" in the preputial sac (therefore the state is markedly less frequent in circumcised persons). Infections of the vaginal mucosa constitute an additional source.

b) *Vulvovaginitis candidamycetica.* One form occurred in younger women (average age 22 years), 70 per cent of whom took ovulation inhibitors; 14 per cent were pregnant and 5 per cent had an additional trichomoniasis. The other form occurred in older women (average age 55 years), who had mostly local anomalies of the uterus (prolapse, carcinoma, status post carcinoma, status post x-ray treatment); sometimes general diseases like diabetes. See Fig. 5.

Origin of yeast and pathogenesis: saprophytes of mucous membranes becoming parasitic by anatomic or endocrinologic anomalies (retention of secretion, raised glycogen content of the epithelium (*Seeliger and Vögtle-Junkert, 1975*). Because of the extremely active formation of "germ tubes" by the mycetes, a possible hormonal stimulation of the mycotic growth is presumed.

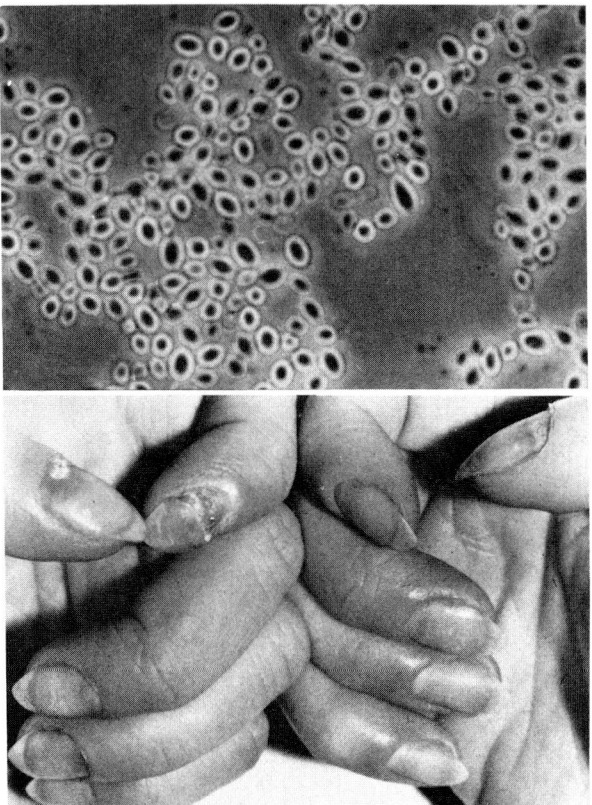

Fig. 6. Paronychia mycetica in a children's nurse, having the same clinical appearance as a *Candida* paronychia. Causative yeast (right hand side) *Torulopsis glabrata.* × 480.

B) Forms affecting mainly the nails, especially the paronychium (*paronychia candidamycetica*)

1) *Paronychia candidamycetica adultorum*

Occurs almost only on the fingers of persons having close contact with infants and rinsing their diapers (Fig. 6). Their average age is 40 years, and the sex incidence, m:f = 8:92.

Epidemiologically and pathogenically, the same applies to CA of the finger webs. Both conditions often occur together. The nail fold is particularly favourable for colonization of yeasts by damage to the natural sealing barrier in manicure and retention of moisture in the area where even single spores can survive

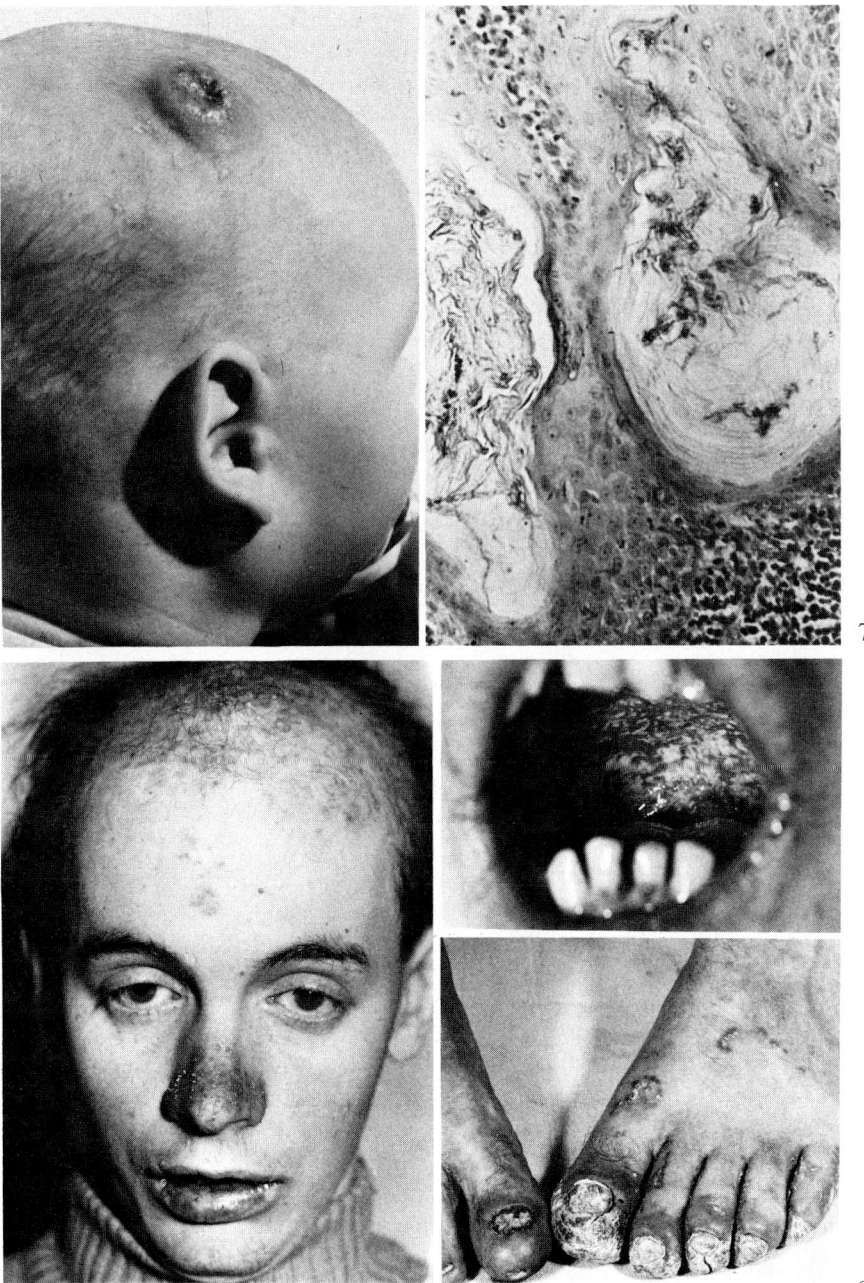

and multiply. Pathogenesis: beside the physico-chemical factors already mentioned, cold-induced angiospasms with reduction of tissue metabolism and hence of the local defence mechanism and extreme abundance of yeasts.

Other persons highly exposed to infection are laundry workers and bar personnel and those who work with fruit and meat. Here women are employed in almost the same number as men. The yeasts are often present in combination with bacteria (*cocci, B. pyocyaneum*).

2) *Paronychia candidamycetica neonatorum (praematurum)*

Occurs frequently in premature infants; 70 per cent of markedly immature infants are affected. Usually other body regions like oral mucosa, intertriginous areas, fingers and toes are involved, contrary to the form seen in adults. This is evidence that a general and not only a local reduced resistance exists, probably because of the prematureness of these infants. The lesions heal spontaneously after some weeks. This never occurs in paronychias of adults.

C) Forms affecting mainly the hair system (*folliculitis candidamycetica*)

Hairs are very seldom affected by yeasts; we have encountered only 12 cases.

1) *Acute purulent folliculitis form*

Occurs mainly in adults, especially men (beard areas). Pathogenesis: local pre-existing lesions, i.e. by herpes simplex (*Meinhof,* 1970; *Male,* 1973) or bacterial infections (*Staib et al.,* 1975). There may be a steroid effect.

2) *Primarily chronic, oligophlegmasic granulomatous form*

Occurs extremely seldom, almost exclusively in infants (first and second trimester of life) and young children, generally with a marked CA of the oral mucosa and the nails also. There are two variants (Table I/III/4; Figs. 7, 8): one occurring chiefly in the first weeks of life and caused by congenital, usually hereditary immunopathies, having almost always a fulminating course and a bad prognosis. The other type appears usually later and is more probably the consequence of endocrinopathies. It tends to be chronic and in most cases has good healing chances (*Higgs and Wells,* 1974; *Meinhof,* 1975; *Ottolenghi,* 1975).

Fig. 7. Candida granuloma in the right parietal region in a case of acute mucocutaneous candidosis in a 10 week-old boy suffering from a severe congenital immunopathy (combined with "BCG-itis"). Histological features (right): hair follicles and hairs destroyed. PAS staining, × 160.

Fig. 8. Chronic mucocutaneous candidosis in a patient suffering from acrodermatitis enteropathica.

References

Auger, P. and Jeannine Joly: Etude de quelques aspects de la pathogenese des infections à *Candida albicans,* Sabouraudia *13:* 263–273 (1975).
Blaschke-Hellmessen, R.: Mund- und Hautsoor, seltene Candidamykosen bei Säuglingen und Kleinkindern?, Dtsch. Gesund Wes. *26:* 1323–1327(1971).
Bernhardt Hannelore: Zum Vorkommen von Hefepilzen im Magen des Menschen, mykosen *11* (11): 799–906 (1968).
Bernhardt Hannelore: Untersuchungen zur Hefebesiedelung des Menschen, Zbl. Hyg. I. Abt. Orig. *223:* 244–254 (1973).
Catterali, R.D.: Candida albicans and the contraceptive pill, Lancet II, 468–830 (1966).
Chen, T.Y. and Webster, J.H.: Oral monilia. Study on patients with head and neck cancer during radiotherapy, Cancer (Philad.) *34/2:* 246–249 (1974).
Chotiner, H.C. and Piver, M.S.: Monilia septicemia associated with hyperalimentation, Obstet-Gynec. N.Y. *38:* 896–898 (1971).
Curry, C.R. and Quie, P.G.: Fungal septicemia in patients receiving parenteral hyperalimentation, New Engl. J. Med. *285:* 1221–1225 (1971).
Daniel, W.: Mögliche Ursachen von Candida-Mykosen im Bereich des weibl. Genitales, Ärztl. Prax. *24/12,* 549–552 (1972).
Dennis, D.L.; Peterson, C.G. and Fletcher, W.S.: Candida septicemia in the severely traumatized patient, J. Trauma *8:* 177–185 (1968).
Dourov, N. and Dustin, P.: Fréquence des mycoses dans les hématopathies malignes traitées, Ann. Soc. Belge Méd. Trop. *44:* 909–930 (1964).
Drouhet, E.: Traitement des infections mycosiques à *Candida albicans* par un nouvel antibiotique antifongique, Bull. Inst. Pasteur *70:* 391–464 (1972).
Gonzáles-Mendoza, A. and Aguirre-Garcia, J.: Mycoses dues à des champignons opportunistes observées au cours de 1000 autopsies, Sabouraudia *5:* 341–349 (1967).
Higgs, Janet M. and Wells, R.S.: Klassifizierung der chronischen muco-cutanen Candidiasis mit Betrachtung zum klinischen Bild und zur Therapie, Hautarzt *25:* 159–165 (1974)
Huhn, F.O.: Candidaperitonitis. Lebensbedrohliche Organmanifestation der Soormykose nach langfristiger Antibioticabehandlung, Med. Klin. *66:* Nr. 41 (1971).
Kecht, B.: Candida-Sepsis, Wr. Klin. Wschr. Jg. 85, Heft *33/34:* 549–553 (1973).
Kozinn, Ph.J. and Taschdjian, C.L.: The precipitin test in systemic candidiasis, J. Amer. med. Ass. *198:* 170–173 (1966).
Lachenicht, Ph. and Potel, J.: Extragenitale Sprosspilzinfektionen und ihre Bedeutung für die Frauenheilkunde, Med. Klin. *66:* No. 38, 1273–1277 (1971).
Law, E.J.; Kim, O.J.; Stieritz, D.D., and MacMillan, B.G.: Experience with systemic candidiasis in the burned patient, J. Trauma *12:* 543–552 (1972).
Lehner, T. and Ward, R.G.: Iatrogenic oral candidosis, Brit. J. Derm. *83:* 161–166 (1970).
Lehrer, R.I. and Cline, M.J.: Leukocyte myeloperoxydase deficiency and disseminated candidiasis: the role of myeloperoxydase in resistance to *Candida* infection, J. clin. Invest. *48:* 1478–1488 (1969).
Lipnik, M.J.; Kligman, A.M., and Strauss, R.: Antiobiotics and fungous Infections, J. Invest. Dermat. *18:* 247–249 (1952).
Louria, D.B.; Greenberg, S.M., and Molander, D.W.: Fungemia caused by certain nonpathogenic strains of the family cryptococcaceae, New Engl. J. Med. *263:* 1281–1284 (1960).
Louria, D.B.; Blevins, A.; Armstrong, D.; Burdick, R., and Liebermann, P.: Fungemia caused by "nonpathogenic" yeasts, Arch. intern. Med. *119:* 247–252 (1967).
MacMillan, B.G.; Law, E.J., and Holder, I.A.: Experience with *Candida* infections in the burn patient, Arch. Surg. *104:* 509–514 (1972).

Male, O.: Über aktuelle Probleme in der Mykologie, Wr. Klin. Wschr. *24:* 442–445 (1964).
Male, O.: Zur allergenen Wirksamkeit saprophytischer Sprosspilze des Intestinaltraktes, In: Krankheiten durch Aktinomyzeten und verwandte Erreger. Wechselwirkung zwischen pathogenen Pilzen und Wirtsorganismus. S. 102–107 (Springer-Verlag, Berlin-Heidelberg-New York 1967).
Male, O.: Vergleichende Untersuchungen über das enzymatische Verhalten dermatotroper und nichtdermatotroper Myzeten, Zbl. Bakt. I. Abt. Orig. *217:* 111–127 (1971).
Male, O.: Zur Pathogenese und Epidemiologie der superfiziellen Candidiasis, Derm. Wschr. *159:* 400–402 (1973a).
Male, O.: Pilzkrankheiten. In: Spezielle pathologische Anatomie. Bd. 7 (Hrg. W. Doerr, G. Seifert, E. Uehlinger, 57–111 (Springer-Verl. Berlin-Heidelberg–New York 1973b).
Marget, W., und Schwab, J.: Candida albicans. Ein Beispiel für "opportunistisch pathogene" Krankheitserreger, Münch. med. Wschr. *113:* No. 49, 1637 (1971).
Meinhof, W.: Zum Krankheitsbild der Folliculitis barbae candidomycetica, Hautarzt *21:* 312–318 (1970).
Meinhof, W.: Angeborene Immundefektsyndrome und Candida-Mykosen, Canesten-Symposium 5–8. Juni, München, 1975.
Mirsky, H.S. and Cuttner, J.: Fungal infections in acute leukemia, Cancer *30:* 348–352 (1960)
Mobacken, H. and Lindholm, L.: Chronic mucocutaneous candidiasis, dermatophytosis and defective cellular immunity on monocygotic twins, Acta Derm. Venerol. (Stockh.) *54/3:* 203–208 (1974).
Montes, L.F.; Pittmann, C.S.; Moore, W.J.; Taylor, C.D., and Cooper, M.D.: Chronic mucocutaneous candidiasis. Influence of thyroid status, JAMA, Vol. *221:* No. 2 10 (1972).
Ottolenghi, F.; Andreassi, L.; Sbano, E., und Fimiani, M.: Diffuse chronische mucocutane Candidosis: Das Verhalten der isolierten *Candida* gegenüber Antibiotica *in vitro,* Hautarzt *26:* 260–263 (1975).
Rayner, C.R.W.: Disseminated-candidiasis in a severely burned patient, Plast. reconstr. Surg. *51:* 461–463 (1973).
Rieth, H., und Wildfeuer, A.: Parasitische Pilze im Intestinaltrakt, ihre Verschleppung insbesondere in den Genitalbereich und neue Möglichkeiten zu ihrer Bekämpfung, Castellania *4* (1) 7–10 (1976).
Schirar, A.; Rendu, C.; Vielh, J.P., and Gautray, J.P.: Congenital mycosis (*Candida albicans*), Biol. neonate (Basel) *24/5–6:* 273–288 (1974).
Scholer, H.J.: Diagnose der Hefemykosen innerer Organe. Candidiasis und Cryptococcose, Therap. Umschau *31:* Heft 6, 402–409 (1974a).
Scholer, H.J.: Stellung und Bedeutung der Mykosen unter den menschlichen Infektionskrankheiten, Path. Microbiol. *41:* 199–231 (1974b).
Seebacher, C.: Zur Pathogenese der Dermatitis seborrhoides infantum. Dtsch. Ges. wesen 27, H. *52:* 2477–2481 (1972).
Seelig, M.S.: Mechanisms by which antibiotics increase the incidence and severity of candidiasis and alter the immunological defenses, Bact. Rev. Vol. *30:* Nr. 2, 442–459 (1966).
Seeliger, H.P.R., und Ute Vögtle-Junkert: Die Candidamykose. Epidemiologie, Ursache und Therapie, Dtsch. Ärztebl.-Ärztl. Mitt. *16:* 1119–1123 (1975).
Staib, F.; Grosse, G., and Mishra, S.K.: Staphylococcus aureus and *Candida albicans* infection, Proceed. of ISHAM, Tokyo, 1975 pp. 85–86.
Vust, J.F. et Grigoriu, D.: Les candidoses septicémiques chez les brûlés, Schweiz. med. Wschr. *103:* 481–484 (1973).
Winner, H.I., and Hurley, R.: Candida albicans. (Churchill & Co., London, 1964).

Prof. Dr. *O. Male,* 1st Dermatological University Clinic, Medical School, *Vienna* (Austria)

Mycotoxins and Abnormal Fetal Development

A. Abramovici

Tel-Aviv University, Sackler School of Medicine and Beilinson Hospital, Petah-Tiqva

Introduction

Mycotoxins are secondary metabolites of fungi, which can induce toxic reactions in the living organism. Small quantities of such toxins, when ingested, inhaled, or on contact, are able to induce a variety of symptoms which sometimes form well identified entities. From the earliest times it is known that contamination of edible food or grains by parasitic fungi can cause disaster to entire communities. As early as 600 B.C., an Assyrian bas-relief alludes to "noxious pustules in the ear of grain," while the ancient Greeks were reluctant to eat the "black maladorous product of Macedonia" which was the infested rye.

In the Middle Ages, written records appeared concerning strange and uncontrollable epidemics of gangrene of the extremities and convulsions, symptoms which are now identifiable as ergot poisoning. The oxytocic effect of ergotoxin on the pregnant womb, which increases the chances of abortion, was used by midwives long before it was adopted in obstetrics.

Another kind of mycotoxicosis epidemic called "aleukia" emerged during the third decade of this century in the Ukraine; it decimated horses as well as man. This disease, characterized by extensive hemorrhages, followed the consumption of bread made from grains infested by *Fusarium* species.

During the last twenty years, great progress has been made in the identification of the chemical nature and on the purification of mycotoxins from various molds. Paralleling these efforts, research has been undertaken to elucidate their possible effects in various experimental animals. For more detailed information on biosynthetic pathways and the biological effects of mycotoxins, the reader is referred to recent comprehensive reviews (*Austwick*, 1975; *Ciegler et al.*, 1971; *Kadis et al.*, 1971; *Purchase*, 1974; *Wogan*, 1975).

Species-specific tolerance and organ-specific vulnerability render the pathogenic idiosyncrasy to mycotoxins different in various animals. The liver and kidneys seem to be most susceptible organs, while the brain and dermal tissues are affected to a lesser degree. Some mycotoxins such as aflatoxin B_1 and sterigmatocystin are well known to possess a carcinogenic effect on the liver as well as a damaging effect on proliferating cells (*Enomoto and Saito,* 1972).

In spite of the large accumulation of data on the pathogenic effects of mycotoxins in adult animals, there is only sparce evidence of their possibly noxious effect on developing embryonic tissues or organs. Embryonated eggs were used in the past for toxicological studies of these compounds; but this method has been applied rather in the search for cheaper and more convenient ways to culture the fungi than to study their embryotoxicity (*Moore,* 1943; *Buddingh,* 1952; *Lafont and Frayssinet,* 1969).

It should be emphasized that the effects of mycotoxins are perceptible only after long periods of successive exposures; but such conditions are not encountered in teratological experiments. The classical concept of dysmorphogenesis is commonly linked to more acute conditions which act at definite sensitive periods of development, thus interfering with normal organogenesis. In these terms, the efficiency of an agent will depend on its pharmacokinetic properties at a given period. Thus, the paucity of data on the effects of mycotoxins on developing embryos is hardly surprising. We review here the current state of knowledge on possible ways whereby mycotoxins can interfere with normal fetal development.

Embryolethal and Teratogenic Effects

The embryotoxic effect of mycotoxins was studied in almost all the cases cited using pure chemical compounds rather than crude extracts. In Table I, the main compounds tested, or reported incidentally to possess some embryotoxic characteristics, are listed alphabetically according to their origin.

I. *Aflatoxins*

Aflatoxins are the largest group of mycotoxins; they are produced by many fungi, including a number of *Aspergillus spp.,* but mainly by *A. flavus* from whence the name derives. These fungi infest many vegetables and cereals as well as meat and other dairy products. Chemically, these toxins are highly substituted coumarins and contain a fused dihydrofuran configuration. They have a hepatotoxic effect and are some of the most powerful carcinogens among the mycotoxins (*Detroy et al.,* 1971).

The first indication of a teratogenic effect of aflatoxin was reported by *Verrett et al.* (1964), in chick embryos treated at very early stages of development. Among the malformations encountered, the limbs were mostly affected; however the eyes and other head structures are also vulnerable (*Verrett et al.,* 1964; *Bassir and Adekunle,* 1970a). The embryonic response depends on the developmental stage; thus at younger stages the embryos are more susceptible than are the older embryos (*Bassir and Adekunle,* 1970a, b). Administration of small doses of aflatoxin at early stages is more disastrous than higher doses at later stages of development (*Detroy et al.,* 1971). On the other hand, the dose response is also determined by the route of administration of aflatoxin. Malformations were induced when the compound was injected into the yolk sac (*Bassir and Adekunle,* 1970a); administration of this compound via the air chamber of the egg was devoid of any teratogenic effect (*Lafont and Frayssinet,* 1969). This difference may be explained on the basis that the air chamber at this early stage of development, contrary to the yolk sac, does not have any vascular system. Therefore, the passive presence of the compound may not be teratogenically effective — it must be also absorbed and carried into the embryonic body through the blood stream. It was also reported that aflatoxin can induce growth retardation in chick embryos, independent either of the period or the mode of administration of aflatoxin (*Lafont and Frayssinet,* 1969; *Bassir and Adekunle,* 1970a).

Among the mammalian embryos, those of hamsters are the most susceptible. Injected into the pregnant female on the eighth day of gestation, aflatoxin B_1 induces malformations in the head region of the fetus in addition to having a high lethal effect (*di Paolo et al.,* 1967). The mouse embryo and to a certain extent the rat are both more resistant to the teratogenic effect of aflatoxin than the hamster embryo (*di Paolo et al.,* 1967; *Buttler and Wigglesworth,* 1966). Aflatoxin appears also without effect on swine reproduction, the litter size being normal and without microscopically detectable lesions (*Hintz et al.,* 1967). Such a response variability among species is a well known phenomenon in the behaviour of many teratogenic agents. Resistance in the mouse to aflatoxin effects may be attributed to a faster rate of toxin degradation in the adult mouse liver (*Enomoto and Saito,* 1972), thus implicitly reducing its transfer rate through the placenta.

In addition to its lethal and teratogenic potency, aflatoxin B_1 can also induce pathological lesions in the liver of chick embryos (*Bassir and Adekunle,* 1970b) as well as in hamster embryos (*di Paolo et al.,* 1967). These lesions are characterized by focal areas of fatty changes together with some proliferation of the reticulo-endothelial cells. Such a hepatotoxic activity might be regarded as an incipient phase in the genesis of cirrhotic and/or carcinogenic lesions observed in adult animals after aflatoxin treatment (*Wogan,* 1975).

The possibility that the lethal effect at early stages of development in the mammalian embryo may result from a previous reaction of the toxin with gametogenesis must also be considered. It is known that tissues with a high proliferative rate are more susceptible to aflatoxin toxicity (*Enomoto and Saito,* 1972). This may be the explanation for the atrophy of testes together with azospermia that occurs in treated rats (*Richir et al.,* 1965). It is worthwhile also

Table I. Embryotoxic and teratogenic effects of mycotoxins

Mycotoxin	Fungus species	Host species	Germ cells & implantation	Embryonic lethality	Teratogenicity and time of administration	Miscellaneous embryopathies	References
Aflatoxin B_1; G_0	*Aspergillus flavus*	chick embryo	—	+	limbs, head, eyes, roughness of feathers (1st day of incubation)	hepatomegalia, liver fatty changes, growth retardation	*Verrett et al.* (1964) *Bassir and Adekunle* (1970), *Lafont and Frayssinet* (1969)
		hamster	—	+	CNS (8th day of gestation)	hepatic injuries growth retardation	*di Paolo et al.* (1967)
		mouse	—	+	—	—	*di Paolo et al.* (1967)
		rat	testicular atrophy, azospermia	—	—	growth retardation	*Butler and Wigglesworth* (1966) *Richir et al.* (1965)
		swine	—	—	—	—	*Hintz et al.* (1967)
Ergot alkaloids Ergotoxin	*Claviceps purpurea*	human and other mammalian	oxytocic	+	—	ergotism	*Goodman and Gilman* (1970)
Lysergic acid derivates	Synthetic	human and other mammalian	chromosomal aberations (?)	rat mice	controversial	—	*Dishotsky et al.* (1971)
Kojic acid	*Aspergillus spp.* *Penicillium spp.*	chick embryo	—	+	—	—	*Wilson* (1971a)
Mycophenolic acid	*Penicillium stoloniferum* *Penicillium brevi-compactum*	rat	implantation failure	+	—	—	*Wilson* (1971b)
Ochratoxin A	*Aspergillus ochraceus*	rat	—	+	—	—	*Still et al.* (1971)
		mouse	—	+	cranio-facial (8th day of gestation)	—	*Hood et al.* (1976)

Patulin	*Aspergillus clavatus* *Penicillium patulum*	salamander	mitotic spindle and chromosomal aberations in eggs	+	—	*Sentein* (1955)
Rubratoxin B	*Penicillium rubrum* *Penicillium purpurogenum*	mouse	—	+	head, eyes, cleft palate, umbilical hernia (10–12th day of gestation)	Growth retardation	*Hood et al.* (1973)
Sterigmatocystin	*Aspergillus versicolor* *Aspergillus flavus*	chick embryo	—	+	limbs (5th day of incubation)	Growth retardation	*Schroeder and Kelton* (1975)
Streptozotocin	*Streptomyces achromogenes*	rat	infertility (chronic effect)	+	—	Growth retardation Hyperglycemia Hypoinsulinemia Placental lesions	*Golob* (1969) *Sybulski and Maugham* (1972) *Prager et al.* (1974) *Liban et al.* (1976)
Trichothecene compounds: T₂ toxin	*Fusarium* spp.	chick embryo mouse	— —	— +	feathers tail and limbs (10th day of gestation)	— —	*Wyatt et al.* (1975) *Hood et al.* (1976)
Fusarenon X	*Fusarium nivale* *Fusarium tricinctum*	rat	impaired spermatogenesis	—	—	—	*Enomoto and Saito* (1972)
Zearalenone (F₂ toxin)	*Fusarium graminearum*	swine	estrogenic effect	+	limbs	—	*Mirocha et al.* (1971) *Miller et al.* (1973)
	Fusarium culmorum	mouse rat	estrogenic effect	—	—	—	*Mirocha et al.* (1971)

to mention that long term administration is devoid of any significant effect through three generations of rat offsprings (*Alfin-Slater et al.*, 1969); the toxin is not transmitted into the eggs of hens (*Kratzer et al.*, 1969) when the latter are given very high doses of aflatoxin. The number of eggs laid by such hens was normal although there was a decrease in the rate of their hatchability.

II. *Miscellaneous* Aspergillus *Mycotoxins*

Several species of *Aspergillus* are able to synthesise other types of toxins which have a close structural relationship to aflatoxin B_1, and are considered as coumarin substitutes.

A. *Ochratoxins.* Ochratoxins are a group of metabolites produced mainly by *A. ochraceus* growing on corn, wheat and barley. There are two types of this toxin; the type A is twice as nephrotoxic to rats and ducklings as type B (*Steyn*, 1971). Ochratoxin A given *per os* to pregnant rats on the tenth day of gestation induces a high percent of fetal death and embryonic resorption (*Still et al.*, 1971). The ground extract of this compound is embryolethal to the same extent as the purified form, while its hydrolytic derivate (dihydroisocoumarin) was found to be inactive at the doses utilized (*Still et al.*, 1971). Teratogenic activity of ochratoxin A has been reported in mice embryos treated on the 8th day of development (*Hood et al.*, 1976) and consisted of cranio-facial malformations.

B. *Sterigmatocystin.* This is a metabolite of *A. versicolor* as well as of other *Aspergillus* strains growing on maize and peanuts. Known to induce hepatoma in several mammalian species (*Enomoto and Saito*, 1972), its effect on reproduction is unknown. Recently, it was reported by *Schroeder and Kelton* (1975) that it possesses a high lethal as well as growth retardation effect when administered to five day old chick embryos. Its teratogenic effect is inconsistent and among the few abnormalities observed, "twisted feet" (arthrogryposis) is the most common.

III. Penicillium *Mycotoxins*

A large number of mycotoxins have been identified from this species but only two compounds were reported to interfere with embryonic development.

A. *Rubratoxin B.* This is an anhydride of glauconic acid produced by many species of *Penicillium*, especially by *P. rubrum* and *P. purpurogenum.* It shows hepatotoxic activity in domestic animals accompanied by hemorrhagic diathesis. Administered to pregnant mice, rubratoxin B has a high lethal effect on young embryos, and a lesser effect when administered at more advanced stages of gestation (*Hood et al.*, 1973). Teratogenic activity was also demonstrated and consisted of various anomalies of the head and eyes as well as cleft palate and umbilical hernia.

B. *Mycophenolic Acid.* This is a metabolic intermediate synthesised by *P. stoloniferum* and *P. brevi-compactum.* Its antibiotic activity was known long before its structure was determined. During its toxicological characterization, it was noted, incidentally, that treated female rats become infertile probably due to an implantation failure of the zygote (*Wilson*, 1971b).

IV. *Mycotoxins of both* Penicillium *and* Aspergillus spp.

During the purification and identification stages, it became evident that some mycotoxins can be synthesised by several different species. The cause and nature of this kind of chemical mimicry is unknown.

A. *Kojic Acid.* This is a hydroxy-pyranone synthesised by several microorganisms (fungi and bacteria) during the fermentation processes of some traditional oriental food. It possesses antibacterial activity and most investigations have been concerned solely with the side effects of this compound in treated animals. When injected into the chorio-alantoic membrane of twelve day old chick embryos, it is 100 percent lethal (*Wilson*, 1971a). However no intoxication in man or animals has been reported after ingestion of food contaminated by this compound.

B. *Patulin.* This is synthesised by many microorganisms and fungi, among them *P. patulum* and *A. clavatus*, growing during the fermentation processes of rotting apples and malted barley (*Ciegler et al.*, 1971). Chemically, it is a lactone derivate of kojic acid. Many biological trials have shown that patulin possesses a marked antibacterial and antifungal activity, while in animals it has a neurotoxic effect (*Ciegler et al.*, 1971). Fertilized eggs of salamander treated with patulin failed to attain further steps in their metamorphosis due to alterations in the mitotic spindle and chromosomal fragmentation (*Sentein*, 1965).

V. *Ergot Alkaloids*

This group of toxins are of historical interest only because of the ergotism endemics which occured since early times. The toxins are produced by *Claviceps purpurea* growing on rye and, chemically, they are all amine derivates of lysergic acid. Few investigations regarding crude extracts of these fungi are concerned with aspects of reproduction. Oxytocic effects on the uteri of women and animals in pregnancy are well known (*Goodman and Gilman*, 1970). The increased motor activity of uterine muscle fibers together with a vaso-constrictive effect may explain the increased risk of abortions characterising this kind of toxicosis. Ergotoxin injected intraperitoneally to rats during the 2nd half of their gestation period was not necessarily embryolethal, but did induce oligogalactia which subsequently brought about a loss of weight in the newborns, during the suckling period (*Sommer and Buchanan*, 1955). There are no data available on possible teratogenic effects of ergotoxin or ergotism poisoning. On the other hand, the effect of lysergic acid diamine (L.S.D.) on reproduction is better documented, although reports are controversial. Possible biological side effects of the compound, including effects on reproduction have been queried. In an extensive survey of the literature on possible genetic damage due to L.S.D. it was concluded that moderate doses do not produce detectable genetic or teratogenic effects in man, or in the animals tested (*Dishotsky et al.*, 1971). Of the latter, mouse embryos seem to be the most susceptible; L.S.D. induced in them malformations of the central nervous system and of the lens. However, the early reports concerning teratogenicity due to L.S.D. demonstrated in hamster and rat embryos have not been further confirmed (*Dishotsky et al.*, 1971).

VI. Fusarium *Mycotoxins*

Strains of *Fusarium spp.* growing on many cereals are able to synthesize (even under unfavorable conditions) various mycotoxins which can be classified in two main chemical groups.

A. *Trichothecenes.* These are closely related to sesquiterpenes, and contain five different radicals which by their interplay offer a large spectrum of compounds. Some of these toxins possess antibacterial, antiviral and even antifungal activity. Among their many biological effects on adult animals, these mycotoxins are known to affect tissues with a high proliferative rate as well as to induce dermatitic phenomena (*Bamburg and Strong*, 1971). Some reports on their effect on reproduction can be related to these actions. Thus Fusarenon X impairs rat spermatogenesis (*Enomoto and Saito*, 1972), while T_2 toxin injected into one day old chickens was found to induce abnormal feather formation (*Wyatt et al.*, 1975). Teratogenic activity of T_2 toxin has been repoted in mice embryos treated on the 10th day of gestation, affecting limbs and the tail (*Hood et al.*, 1976).

B. *Zearalenone or F_2 Toxin.* This is an alkyl derivate of β resorcylic acid, known to have an estrogen-like activity in many animals, including swine, rodents and turkey (*Mirocha et al.*, 1971). First discovered in swine, the effects of this toxin are manifested by uterine edematic enlargement with vaginal prolapse and shrunken ovaries, while pregnant animals may abort. Another expression of estrogenic phenomena was observed in male pigs which developed gynecomasty and testicular atrophy (*Mirocha et al.*, 1971). The abortive effect on pregnant swine, which was at first misinterpreted as a superimposed infection, is now recognised (*Mirocha et al.*, 1971) to be a result of the estrogenic effect of the F_2 toxin. This toxin has a hypomorphic effect on pig fetuses as well as causing increased neonatal mortality (*Miller et al.*, 1973). Some of the piglets showed also non-coordination of hind limb movements. Considered to be excreted with the milk, this toxin reaches the developing newborn, thus contributing to a further deterioration of its health condition.

VII. *Streptozotocin*

Streptozotocin is a glucose nitrosurea compound isolated from *Streptomyces achromogenes*; it is considered to have a wide range of antibiotic activity (*Rerup*, 1970). Concomitantly, it has a diabetogenic effect in rats, characterized by constant hyperglycemic values as a consequence of cytotoxic damage of the β cells of the pancreas (*Rerup*, 1970). The effect of streptozotocin on reproduction was studied only using a morphometric approach; the placentae of the diabetic rats were heavier than normal, while the litter size was normal but hypomorphic (*Golob* 1969; *Prager et al.*, 1974; *Sybulski and Maugham*, 1972). In spite of the growth retardation, no teratogenic effect was observed. The placentae of treated animals showed cystic degeneration in the spongiosa region with accumulation of some carbohydrate deposits ranging from acid mucopolysaccharides and glycogen to glucose (*Liban et al.*, 1976). It is worthwhile noting that the labyrinth region of the placenta remained normal. The severity of placental lesions was more marked, the shorter the lapse of time between administration of a single dose and mating. Fecundity did not seem to be affected by the shorter lapse period; however, chronically treated rats lost their mating ability and died spontaneously in 5–6 months (*Liban et al.*, 1976). The maternal hyperglycemic state is more pronounced than that of the offspring (*Liban et al.*, 1976), supporting the assumption that the placenta can play a homeostatic role in the defence mechanism against diabetes during pregnancy.

Possible Modes of Action of Mycotoxins during Embryogenesis

As previously noted, the various potential effects of some mycotoxins on normal embryonic development can be related to their heterogeneous origin, as well as to their chemical nature. Information is lacking that would permit us to define a typical specific target action for a given toxin. Data quoted in some reports were incidental findings, while in others there are only allusions to, especially, the morpho-pathological aspects. It is tempting to try to assemble the fragmented data into an ontogenetic pattern of the possible modes of action of mycotoxins during embryogenesis. The fetal outcome can be affected at any one of the development stages, starting from gametogenesis, to the suckling period.

I. *Direct Effect on Parental Gametes*

The earliest stage at which mycotoxins are able to interfere with embryonic development is during germ cell formation. During the reproduction period of an adult animal this process is a continuous but very labile one, and can be affected by various factors. Impaired function of gonads may thus originate either as a result of a hormonal imbalance, or through direct interference of toxins with the biosynthesis of nucleic acids during gametogenesis. Zearalenone is the only mycotoxin which has been shown to have an estrogen-like activity in animals (*Mirocha et al.*, 1971). The existence of such hormonal interference may in female animals bring about a change in endometrial receptiveness to implantation of the zygote. The counterpart effect in males is characterized by a feminisation process accompanied by gynecomastia and testicular atrophy, the latter leading to azospermia.

Inhibition of spermatogenesis was also observed after treatment of rats with Fusarenon X (*Enomoto and Saito*, 1972), aflatoxin B_1 (*Richir et al.*, 1965) and T_2 toxin (*Bamburg and Strong*, 1971). Such cytotoxicity towards spermatogonia could be explained at the molecular level by interference with nucleic acids and protein biosynthesis which occurs at high rates in such continuous dividing cells (*Enomoto and Saito*, 1972; *Wogan*, 1975). Aflatoxin is known to inhibit RNA polymerase (*Roy*, 1968) as well as protein synthesis by affecting the polyribosomal stability and the binding capacity of the polyribosomes to endoplastic reticulum membrane in liver cells (*Pong and Wogan*, 1968; *Wogan*, 1975). On the other hand, the trichothecene compounds are considered to act either by inhibition of DNA synthesis (*Bamburg and Strong*, 1971), or by a reduction of protein synthesis also through a polysomal disaggregation mechanism (*Wogan*, 1975).

II. Direct Effect on Embryos

A possible direct effect of some mycotoxins during the early stages of embryonic differentiation was noted among the non-mammalian embryos. Administration of patulin to salamander fertilized eggs brings about complete arrest in their further development (*Sentein*, 1965), while administration of aflatoxins to one day old chick embryos is always accompanied by a high mortality rate in the early stages of development (*Bassir and Adekunle*, 1970a). The extramaternal development of these embryos expose them to high risks of external factors. Besides the hormonal impairment in implantation already mentioned, mammalian embryos are usually not susceptible to teratogenic agents prior to their implantation (*Wilson*, 1967). Most of the dysmorphogenetic response is obtained when the compound is administered during organogenesis, when each organ has its own sensitive period. With this limitation, a number of mycotoxins, such as aflatoxin (*di Paolo et al.*, 1967), ochratoxin A (*Hood et al.*, 1976), rubratoxin B (*Hood et al.*, 1973), T_2 toxin (*Hood et al.*, 1976) and zearalenone (*Mirocha et al.*, 1971; *Miller et al.*, 1973), appear to have a teratogenic effect on several species. The species-specific susceptibility reported in the literature can be imputed to the pharmacokinetic properties of the compounds, concomitant with the existence of an effective process of detoxification in the host. Thus, the chick embryo, which is devoid of maternal protection, is more vulnerable to mycotoxins than is the mammalian embryo. Here, again, we can only speculate on the mode of teratogenic action as being related to interference with nucleic acid and protein synthesis. Fetal growth retardation, usually observed during toxicological assays of mycotoxins, can also be explained in these terms. A fascinating hypothesis concerning dwarfism in chick embryos appearing after aflatoxin administration was advanced by *Bassir and Adekunle* (1970a).

They suggested that the toxin can affect embryonic development via the growth hormone; however no experimental evidence is presented to support this statement. A more likely assumption may be impairment of fetal nutrition as the origin of growth retardation, since this can be linked to maternal health conditions, placental function or even the metabolism of the fetus itself.

The liver of the fetus during its development does not function as efficiently as in the adult, and it is implicit that any morphological damage can interfere with fetal nutrition. It was found that aflatoxin B_1 is able to induce embryonal hepatotoxic injuries in hamsters (*di Paolo et al.*, 1967) and chickens (*Bassir and Adekunle*, 1970b). These lesions were pathologically identical to the incipient phases of liver damage encountered in adult animals (*Detroy et al.*, 1971; *Wogan*, 1975). However, the fetal liver of the mouse (*di Paolo et al.*, 1967) and the rat (*Buttler and Wigglesworth*, 1966) were found to be refractory to aflatoxin action. The pathogenetic pathways in fetal hepatic damage following aflatoxin treatment are not yet elucidated, although an increase in lysosomal enzymes due to a membranal leakage was observed in the livers of several bird embryos treated with aflatoxin (*Adekunle and Elegbe*, 1974).

Histological examination of the placenta after aflatoxin administration does not reveal any pathological lesions in rats (*Buttler and Wigleworth*, 1966), mice, or hamsters (*di Paolo et al.*, 1967). On the other hand, placental lesions were observed in rats treated with streptozotocin prior to mating (*Prager et al.*, 1974; *Liban et al.*, 1976). The presence of these lesions seems to be connected in some way with the homeostatic response of the placenta towards the induced diabetic condition, although the possibility of a primary and direct effect of this toxin on the developing placenta should also be considered.

III. *Indirect Effect on Pregnancy Outcome*

The affinity of some mycotoxins for adult organs such as liver (*Detroy et al.*, 1971), kidney (*Still et al.*, 1971) and leukopoietic tissues (*Bamburg and Strong*, 1971) raises the question whether the maternal health condition influences the intrauterine development of offspring. The establishment of a labile metabolic state in these affected organs could affect the pregnancy outcome in the following ways:

A) Impairment of biosynthetic capabilities of the liver to deal with the supply of essential nutrient materials for the growing fetus.

B) Decreased capacity to detoxify potential noxious agents by the liver or to excrete them as conjugates through the kidney. Thus, the activity of the toxic compound is greater and more likely to affect the embryo.

C) Induced damage to leukopoietic tissues by some trichothecene compounds (*Bamburg and Strong*, 1971) will be expressed by leukopenic and immuno-suppressive effects. Both conditions increase the superimposed risk of infection to the embryo, and the embryolethal effect of the toxin.

Fetal loss is also possible due to the endemic outbreaks of ergotism which have occurred in the past among various mammalian species, including man (*Goodman and Gilman,* 1970). The specific oxytocic effect of ergot alkaloids on uterine contractions, as well as their vasoconstrictive action, increase the rate of abortion in affected animals.

In conclusion, the specific responses of the maternal organism as well as of the fetal tissues and placenta to a mycotoxin are limiting factors which determine whether or not there will be danger to the fetal outcome. The existence of such inadvertent effects, together with lack of criteria for detection and control of mycotoxicoses, necessitates further investigations of such hazards to embryonic development.

References

Adekunle, A.A. and Elegbe, R.A.: Comparative studies on lysosomal activities in mycotoxin treated bird embryos. Envir. Physiol. Biochem. *4:* 289–293 (1974).

Alfin-Slater, R.B.; Aftergood, L.; Hernandez, H.J.; Stern, E., and Melnick, D.: Studies on long term administration of aflatoxin to rats. J. Amer. Oil Chem. Soc. *46:* 493–497 (1969).

Austwick, P.K.C.: Mycotoxins. Br. med. Bull. *31:* 222–229 (1975).

Bamburg, J.R. and Strong, F.M.: 12, 13-Epoxytrichothecenes; in *Kadis, Ciegler and Ajl* Bacterial toxins, vol.VII, pp. 207–292 (Academic Press, New York 1971).

Bassir, O. and Adekunle, A.: Teratogenic action of aflatoxin B_1, palmotoxin B_0 and palmotoxin G_0 in the chick embryo. J. Path. *102:* 49–51 (1970a).

Bassir, O. and Adekunle, A.: The histopathological effects of aflatoxin B_1 and the palmotoxins B_0 and G_0 on the liver of developing chick embryo. FEBS Lett. *10:* 198–201 (1970b).

Buddingh, G.H.: Bacterial and mycotic infections of the chick embryos. Ann. N.Y. Acad. Sci. *55:* 282–287 (1952).

Buttler, W.H. and Wigglesworth, J.S.: The effects of aflatoxin B_1 on the pregnant rat. Br. J. exp. Path. *47:* 242–247 (1966).

Ciegler, A.; Kadis, S., and Ajl, S.J.: Microbial toxins, vol. VI: Fungal toxins (Academic Press, New York 1971).

Detroy, R.W.; Lillehoj, E.B., and Ciegler, A.: Aflatoxins and related compounds; in *Ciegler, Kadis and Ajl* Bacterial toxins, vol.VI, pp. 4–178 (Academic Press, New York 1971).

di Paolo, J.A.; Ajl, S.J., and Erwin, H.: Teratogenic response by hamsters, rats and mice to aflatoxin B_1. Nature *215:* 638–639 (1967).

Dishotsky, N.J.; Loughman, W.D.; Mogar, R.E., and Lipscomb, W.R.: LSD and genetic damage. Is LSD chromosome damaging, carcinogenic, mutagenic or teratogenic? Science *172:* 431–440 (1971).

Enomoto, M. and Saito, M.: Carcinogens produced by fungi. A. Rev. Microbiol. *26:* 279–312 (1972).

Golob, E.: Streptozotocin diabetes bei der schwangeren Ratte. Z. Geburtsh. Gynäk. *171:* 18–38 (1969).

Goodman, L.S. and Gilman, A.: The pharmaceutical basis of therapeutics; IVth ed., pp. 897–904 (MacMillan, New York 1970).

Hintz, H.F.; Heitman, H., jr.; Bioth, A.N., and Gagne, W.E.: Effects of aflatoxin on reproduction in swine. Proc. Soc. exp. Biol. Med. *126:* 146–148 (1967).
Hood, R.D.; Innes, J.E., and Hayes, W.A.: Effects of rubratoxin B on prenatal development in mice. Bull. envir. Contam. Toxicol. *10:* 200–207 (1973).
Hood, R.D.; Kuczuk, M.H., and Szczech, G.M.: Prenatal effects in mice of mycotoxins in combination: Ochratoxin A and T_2 toxin. Teratology *13:* 25A (1976).
Kadis, G.; Ciegler, A., and Ajl, S.J.: Microbial toxins, vol VII: Algal and fungal toxins (Academic Press, New York 1971).
Kratzer, F.H.; Bondy, D.; Wiley, M., and Booth, A.N.: Aflatoxin effects in poultry. Proc. Soc. exp. Biol. Med. *131:* 1281–1283 (1969).
Lafont, J. et Frayssinet, C.: Mycotoxines élaborèes par des *Aspergillus.* Leur activité sur l'embryon de poulet. C.r. Séanc. Soc. Biol. *163:* 1362–1364 (1969).
Liban, E.; Abramovici, A.; Sporn, J.; Prager, R., and Laron, Z.: Morphological and biochemical changes in the placenta of streptozotocin-induced diabetic rats. Harefuah *90:* 508–513 (1976).
Miller, J.K.; Hacking, A.; Harrison, J., and Gross, V.J.: Stillbirth, neonatal mortality and small litters in pigs associated with ingestion of *Fusarium* toxins by pregnant sows. Vet. Rec. *93:* 555–559 (1973).
Mirocha, C.J.; Christensen, C.M., and Nelson, G.H.: F_2 (Zearalenone) estrogenic mycotoxins from *Fusarium;* in *Kadis, Ciegler and Ajl* Microbial toxins, vol. VII; pp. 107–138 (Academic Press, New York 1971).
Moore, M.: The chorioallantoic membrane of the developing chick embryo as a medium for the cultivation and histopathological study of pathogenic fungi. Am. J. Path. *17:* 103–120 (1943).
Prager, R.; Abramovici, A.; Liban, E., and Laron, Z.: Histopathological changes in the placenta of streptozotocin-induced diabetic rats. Diabetologia *10:* 89–91 (1974).
Pong, R.S. and Wogan, G.N.: Effects of aflatoxin B_1 on rat polyribosome profile. Fed. Proc. Fed. Am. Socs exp. Biol. *27:* 552 (1968).
Purchase, I.F.H.: Mycotoxins (Elsevier, Amsterdam 1974).
Rerup, C.C.: Drugs producing diabetes through damage of insulin secreting cells. Pharmac. Rev. *22:* 485–518 (1970).
Richir, C.; Martineaud, M.; Toury, J. et Dupin, H.: Sur les effets cancerigenes de régimes contenent des arachides contaminées. C.r. Séanc. Soc. Biol. *158:* 1375–1377 (1965).
Roy, A.K.: Aflatoxin B_1 and *in vitro* RNA synthesis. Fed. Proc. Fed. Am. Socs exp. Biol. *27:* 552 (1968).
Sentein, P.: Alterations du fuseau mitotique et fragmentation des chromosomes par l'action de la patuline sur l'oeuf d'urodèles en segmentation. C.r. Séanc. Soc. Biol. *149:* 1621–1622 (1955).
Schroeder, H.W. and Kelton, W.H.: Production of sterigmatocystin by some species of the genus *Aspergillus* and its toxicity to chicken embryos. Appl. Microbiol. *30:* 589 (1975).
Sommer, A.F. and Buchanan, A.R.: Effects of ergot alkaloids on pregnancy and lactation in the albino rat. Am. J. Physiol. *180:* 296–300 (1955).
Steyn, P.S.: Ochratoxin and other dihydroisocoumarins; in *Ciegler, Kadis and Ajl* Bacterial toxins, vol. VI, pp. 179–285 (Academic Press, New York 1971).
Still, P.E.; MacKlin, A.W.; Ribelin, W.E., and Smalley, E.B.: Relationship of ochratoxin A to fetal death in laboratory and domestic animals. Nature *234:* 563–564 (1971).
Sybulski, S. and Maugham, G.B.: Use of streptozotocin as a diabetic agent in pregnant rats. Endocrinology *89:* 1537–1540 (1972).
Verrett, J.M.; Marliac, J.P., and McLanghlin, J., jr.: The use of chicken embryo in the assay of aflatoxin toxicity. J. Ass. off. agric. Chem. *47:* 1003–1006 (1964).

Wilson, B.J.: Miscellaneous *Aspergillus* toxins; in *Ciegler, Kadis and Ajl* Microbial toxins, vol. VI, pp. 235–250 (Academic Press, New York 1971a).

Wilson, B.J.: Miscellaneous *Penicillium* toxins; in *Ciegler, Kadis and Ajl* Microbial toxins, vol. VI, pp. 460–470 (Academic Press, New York 1971b).

Wilson, J.G.: Embryological considerations in teratology; in *Wilson and Warkany* Teratology. Principles and technics, pp. 251–261 (University of Chicago Press, Chicago 1967).

Wogan, G.N.: Mycotoxins. A. Rev. Pharmacol. *15:* 437–451 (1975).

Wyatt, R.D.; Hamilton, P.B., and Burmeister, H.R.: Altered feathering of chicks caused by T_2 toxin. Poult. Sci. *54:* 1042–1045 (1975).

Dr. A. *Abramovici,* Tel-Aviv University, Sackler School of Medicine and Beilinson Hospital, *Petah-Tiqva* (Israel)

Immunology: Its Value in Diagnosing Systemic Fungal Infections[1]

L. Kaufman

Center for Disease Control, Public Health Service, U.S. Department of Health, Education and Welfare, Atlanta, Ga.

The nonspecific clinical and morphological manifestations of many of the systemic mycotic infections frequently impede their diagnosis; the rapidity with which such a disease is diagnosed depends mainly on the clinician's suspicions that the patient has a mycotic infection. Such suspicions can only be confirmed through the acquisition of either pertinent cultural or histological data. Unfortunately, such data may be difficult or, in some cases, impossible to acquire. Immunological tests have proven to be useful in establishing the presence of deep-seated mycotic infections. I will describe some of these methods and will discuss their diagnostic and prognostic value.

Aspergillosis

The aspergillosis immunodiffusion (ID) test, with standardized precipitinogens obtained from three *Aspergillus sp.*, is diagnostically and prognostically useful (*Coleman and Kaufman, 1972*). At the Center for Disease Control (CDC) we use *A. fumigatus, A. flavus* and *A. niger* precipitinogens prepared from acetone-precipitated 5-week-old Sabouraud dextrose broth cultures. The greatest number of aspergillosis cases are detected by the concurrent use of these antigens. All *Aspergillus* antigens should be checked for the presence of C-substance, which is capable of reacting with the C-reactive protein frequently found in patients with inflammatory diseases and can form a precipitate that may be erroneously interpreted as being caused by *Aspergillus* antibodies.

Only sera that produce a line or lines of identity with a reference serum

---

[1] Use of trade names is for identification only and does not constitute endorsement by the Public Health Service or by the U.S. Department of Health, Education, and Welfare.

from a person with proven aspergillosis or from selected immunized animals, are considered positive in the ID test. The presence of precipitating antibodies, irrespective of the number of precipitin bands or the titer, indicates infection, fungus ball, or allergy due to an *Aspergillus sp.* Allergic bronchopulmonary aspergillosis should be considered in patients with asthma, transient pulmonary infiltrates, and peripheral eosinophilia. Pulmonary aspergilloma or fungus ball occurs when *A. fumigatus* or other *Aspergillus* species colonize pulmonary cavities in patients with tuberculosis, sarcoidosis, or carcinoma. Invasive aspergillosis includes those cases where aspergilli have been shown to actually penetrate tissue. Using the immunodiffusion (ID) test, we have serologically diagnosed 76 of 78 (97%) fungus ball cases with or without tissue invasion, 28 of 44 (68%) cases of invasive aspergillosis, and 21 out of 28 (75%) cases of allergic bronchopulmonary aspergillosis. Although one or two precipitins can be found with any clinical form of aspergillosis, three or more precipitins were invariably associated with either a fungus ball or invasive disease (*Coleman and Kaufman, 1972*).

The ID test, when used with reference sera, is 100% specific. Occasionally, bands of nonidentiy that are associated with aspergillosis cases are detected. These should lead one to suspect aspergillosis, but a specific diagnosis cannot be made if bands of identity are not present. One cause of nonspecific bands is the C-reactive protein that may react with *Aspergillus* precipitinogens. These nonspecific bands, however, will not fuse with the reference lines to give lines of identity. The non-specific lines due to C-reactive protein may be identified and, at the same time, eliminated, by soaking the agar with 5% sodium citrate for 45 minutes before taking the final reading.

In diagnosed cases of aspergillosis, the number of precipitins in a series of sera taken at different stages, or the precipitin titers, provide clues to the course of the disease. A decline in the number of precipitins or in precipitin titers reflects recovery.

Most of the fungus ball and allergic bronchopulmonary case sera do not have to be concentrated to demonstrate precipitin bands. Some unconcentrated sera from invasive cases are precipitin-positive. Unconcentrated precipitin-negative sera from patients suspected of invasive aspergillosis, particularly those who are immunosuppressed, should be retested after the sera have been concentrated three or four times.

Complement-fixation (CF) tests for aspergillosis with filtrate antigens of *A. fumigatus* have been developed and evaluated (*Walter and Jones, 1968; Parker et al., 1970; Young and Bennett, 1971*). Positive reactions demonstrated by titers of 1:8 or higher are considered indicative of infection, colonization, or allergy due to an *Aspergillus* sp. Studies in this laboratory with the CF test indicate that it is less sensitive than the ID test, but it is, nevertheless, sufficiently specific to be useful. All sera from patients with suspected cases of aspergillosis should be tested with a battery of *Aspergillus spp.* antigens.

Blastomycosis

The CF and ID tests are used to detect antibodies to *Blastomyces dermatitidis* (*Kaufman et al.*, 1973). The CF test is limited by the fact that, with the yeast form antigen currently used, it is insensitive and nonspecific. Less than 50% of the sera taken from patients with culturally or histologically proven blastomycosis are positive in the CF test. Heterologous case sera, such as those from patients with coccidioidomycosis, histoplasmosis, and paracoccidioidomycosis, may also react in the CF test when yeast antigens of *B. dermatitidis* are used. Titers of 1:8 or greater are considered presumptive evidence for blastomycosis. In view of the cross-reactions noted with the *B. dermatitidis* antigens, however, only sera exhibiting high or rising titers are regarded as good indicators of blastomycosis.

In addition, sera containing precipitating as well as complement fixing antibodies for *B. dermatitidis* are considered evidence of blastomycosis. Because the CF test is insensitive, a negative reaction does not exclude a diagnosis of active blastomycosis.

The CF test may be used to monitor the effects of therapy in a serologically positive patient diagnosed as having blastomycosis. A reduction in titer or change to negativity usually reflects a favorable prognosis.

The ID test is qualitative, has a sensitivity of about 80%, and is entirely specific when performed with reference sera that contain A and B precipitins. Blastomycosis case sera reacting with yeast-filtrate antigen(s) of *B. dermatitidis* may produce one (A) or two (A and B) precipitin lines. Only sera that produce lines of identity with either of the reference lines are considered positive for blastomycosis. In established cases of blastomycosis, the disappearance of precipitin lines is evidence of a favorable prognosis. We have, however, noted that, in successfully treated patients, such precipitin reactions are not as rapid as the clinical response. We have, for example, demonstrated A or A and B precipitins in cured patients 1 month or longer after treatment has been stopped and symptoms have disappeared.

Coccidioidomycosis

The first immunologic manifestations of coccidioidomycosis are revealed by delayed dermal sensitivity tests. Two antigens are currently used to elicit such reactions: coccidioidin, the classical antigen derived from mycelial culture filtrates, and spherulin, a soluble extract of autolyzed spherules of *Coccoidioides immitis* (*Levine et al.*, 1969).

Serologic tests with coccidioidin are of great value in detecting and monitoring cases of coccidioidomycosis. Any precipitin reaction or CF titer should be considered presumptive evidence of *C. immitis* infection. The tube precipitin test result usually becomes positive during the first month of illness and is most valuable in detecting early primary infection or cases undergoing an exacerbation of existing disease. The test result usually reverts to negative between 1 and 5 months after infection and the test has no prognostic value.

The results of the latex particle agglutination test are considered comparable with those of the tube precipitin test, and the latex test is recommended as a screening procedure. It is more sensitive than the tube precipitin test, but it also yields some false positives (*Huppert et al.*, 1968; *Wallraff*, 1971).

The CF test has both diagnostic and prognostic value. CF titers develop later than precipitin titers, rise in proportion to the severity of the infection, and decline as the patient improves. The CF test detects a high proportion of infections missed by the tube precipitin and latex particle agglutination tests (*Wallraff*, 1971). A qualitative ID test (*Huppert and Bailey*, 1965) has been developed for use as a screening procedure for determining which sera should be tested by the CF test. It gives results that correlate well with those of the CF test. Low CF reactions, i.e., titers of 2 and 4, have been found to be indicative of residual, early, or meningeal coccidioidomycosis (*Smith et al.*, 1950). Such titers, however, are not always of diagnostic significance. Recently, *Kaufman and Clark* (1974) found that 25 of 65 (38%) sera which were positive in the CF test with coccidioidin at titers of 8 or less represented false positive reactions. Studies in my laboratory indicate no cross-reactivity between histoplasmin "H" and "M" antigens, *B. dermatitidis* precipitinogens, and coccidioidin. The parallel use of the CF and ID tests is an effective means for specifically diagnosing coccidioidomycosis in patients with low levels of complement-fixing antibodies. In our routine CF diagnostic services, serum dilutions are initiated at the 1:8 level. We recommend that only sera which are negative for complement-fixing antibodies at 1:8 but positive in the ID test with coccidioidin be selected for titration at the 1:2 and 1:4 levels. Our data indicate that sera positive in the CF test in the 1:2 to 1:8 range and also positive in the ID test reflect active or recent *C. immitis* infections.

Counterelectrophoresis (CEP) appears to provide a reliable and rapid means for detecting (within 90 minutes) *C. immitis* antibodies that are reactive in CF and ID tests. *Kleger and Kaufman* (unpublished data) used a discontinuous buffer system and a gel matrix composed of agarose and ionagar No. 2 (*Kleger and Kaufman*, 1973) to study sera from 10 proven cases of coccidioidomycosis. Identical reactions were obtained in the CEP and ID tests for coccidioidomycosis. Cross-reactions were not noted with sera from 11 persons with histoplasmosis and 1 person with cryptococcosis. As is inherent with ID tests that use crude antigens, the CEP test lacks specificity. When the test is used in conjunction with reference antisera, however, the specificity or lack of specificity of a reaction can be determined.

Smith et al. (1956) considered fixation of complement by cerebrospinal fluid (CSF) to be diagnostic of coccidioidal meningitis. They also found, however, that in approximately 25 percent of patients with coccidioidal meningitis, the CSF did not contain detectable CF antibodies. Using ID- and CF-negative CSF specimens from several patients with coccidioidal meningitis, *Pappagianis et al.* (1972) recently demonstrated specific precipitins in cerebro-spinal fluids (CSF) that had been concentrated and tested by ID. Unfortunately, the detection of precipitins in CSF is not always diagnostic of meningeal coccidioidomycosis. Using the concentration technique, these investigators also detected coccidioidal antibodies in CSF specimens from patients with non-meningeal coccidioidomycosis. Their studies indicated that a positive ID test on a CSF specimen denotes central nervous system infection only when CSF glucose is also decreased and protein and cell levels elevated.

Candidosis

Candidosis is the most common fungus infection affecting the compromised host (*Bodey,* 1966; *Hart et al.,* 1969; *Rifkind et al.,* 1967). In spite of the frequency of such infections and the time devoted to perfecting means of detecting them, pre-mortem diagnoses are very difficult to establish. Many laboratories use immunologic procedures to provide supplemental data which could establish a pre-mortem diagnosis of systemic candidosis in the compromised host and to monitor the course of the disease. Since the pioneering studies of *Stallybrass* (1964) and *Taschdjian et al.* (1964, 1967), who demonstrated precipitins to *Candida albicans* in patients with systemic *Candida sp.* infections, the ID test has become the serologic test most widely used for candidosis. The latter workers found the ID test to be positive in 85% to 90% of cases of systemic candidosis and that it was generically specific.

At CDC we are using ID and latex agglutination (LA) tests with homogenate antigens of *C. albicans* (*Stickle et al.,* 1972). The ID test has a sensitivity of 88%, and the LA test a sensitivity of about 90%, in proven candidosis cases. The ID test is highly specific; extrageneric reactions occur only with *Torulopsis glabrata* antisera. The LA test is less specific, particularly at lower serum dilutions. LA titers of 1:8 or higher appear to have diagnostic value. The LA test offers the opportunity to quantitate antibody responses and, when used concommitantly with the ID test, it provides specific prognostic data.

The detection of precipitins or the recognition of fourfold changes in agglutinin titers are considered presumptive evidence of systemic candidosis. Infection should be seriously considered when serial serum specimens demonstrate serologic conversion or show an increase in the number of precipitins. These reactions, however, can also indicate colonization by *Candida spp.,* transient candidemia, or infection due to *T. glabrata*.

We have noted as many as seven distinct precipitin lines in our ID test with serum from patients with candidosis. Four or more precipitin lines or high LA titers are frequently related to severity of the disease.

Counterelectrophoresis (CEP) tests provide results essentially similar to those of the ID test, but these results are obtained in less time.

Cryptococcosis

Excellent diagnostic and prognostic immunologic procedures are available for studying suspected or proven cases of cryptococcosis. These are the indirect fluorescent antibody (IFA) tests (*Vogel,* 1966) and the tube agglutination (TA) tests (*Gordon and Vedder,* 1966) for *Cryptococcus neoformans* antibodies and the LA test for cryptococcal capsular polysaccharide antigens (*Bloomfield et al.,* 1963). Our experience indicates that the combined use of these three procedures enables the laboratory worker to diagnose cryptococcosis rapidly and accurately (*Kaufman and Blumer,* 1968). Both the IFA and TA tests are performed because their capacity to detect *C. neoformans* antibodies in proven case sera varies – sera that are negative with the IFA test are often positive with the TA test, and *vice versa.* The antibody tests are of value in detecting early or localized cryptococcosis and in indicating prognosis, but are less specific than the LA test. The antibody tests are reactive with less than 50% of the sera from proven cases. The IFA test has a specificity of about 79%, whereas the TA test has a specificity of about 95%.

The LA test is valuable in diagnosing active nonmeningeal and meningeal cryptococcosis, particularly the latter; of 39 patients recently studied with culturally proven meningeal cryptococcosis, 36 (92%) had spinal fluids positive for cryptococcal antigen by the LA test (*Goodman et al.,* 1971). It is more sensitive for diagnosing cryptococcal meningitis than the India ink test. False-positive reactions are rare and occur mostly with some sera from patients with severe rheumatoid arthritis and, less frequently, with a small number of spinal fluid specimens. These do not present a problem, however, since all cryptococcal antigen LA-positive specimens are evaluated by routine checks with latex particles sensitized with rabbit normal (pre-immune) globulin, hitherto referred to as the LN reagent. LA tests in which specimens react with both the latex sensitized with rabbit anti-*C. neoformans* globulins (LI) and LN reagents should be considered equivocal. Such specimens should be titered with both the LI and LN reagents. A fourfold or greater titer obtained with the LI reagent suggests cryptococcosis. A positive reaction in the controlled LA test appears to be highly specific. Increasing titers reflect progressive infections, and declining titers indicate favourable response to chemotherapy and clinical improvement in the patient.

Histoplasmosis

Serologic evidence for histoplasmosis is usually obtained with the CF, ID, and LA tests, either separately or in combination. The most widely used of these procedures is the CF test. Properly performed, it can yield information of diagnostic and prognostic value. Two antigens are used in the CDC's Laboratory Branch Complement Fixation (LBCF) test (*Kaufman et al.,* 1974). One is a suspension of Merthiolate-treated yeast-form cells of *H. capsulatum* (*Schubert and Ajello,* 1957); the other is a soluble mycelial filtrate antigen, histoplasmin (*Harrell et al.,* 1970). These antigens are commercially available (Microbiological Associates, Bethesda, Md.). The CF test with both antigens is very sensitive and has been positive with sera from 96% of the culturally proven cases of histoplasmosis studied (*Kaufman,* 1970). The currently available antigens, however, are not entirely specific. Cross-reactions may occur with sera from patients with blastomycosis, coccidioidomycosis, and other fungal infections. The CF test with the yeast-form antigen has the greatest sensitivity (94%). Consequently, this antigen should be used in the diagnostic laboratory, and where possible, it should be supplemented with either the ID or CEP tests with histoplasmin. The latter tests are useful in examining anticomplementary sera, and, because of their greater specificity, they permit a more accurate diagnosis with those sera that cross-react in CF tests. About 85% of the histoplasmosis case sera can be detected with the ID and CF tests with histoplasmin.

The histoplasmin LA test kit is available commercially (Colab Laboratories, Inc.). This test measures antibody which rises relatively early in the acute phase of histoplasmosis. The test has certain limitations, however: it is frequently negative with sera from persons with chronic histoplasmosis (*Bennett,* 1966) and yields many false positive reactions at low serum dilutions.

CF antibodies in primary pulmonary infections generally are detected 2 to 4 weeks after infection or frequently by the time symptoms appear. They are usually antibodies to the yeast-form antigens. Antibodies to histoplasmin usually develop later in primary pulmonary cases, and titers are generally lower than those with yeast antigens. Because cross-reactions or nonspecific reactions may occur with either antigen, CF results can be difficult to interpret, particularly when the titers are 1:8 and 1:16. Many sera, however, from patients with culturally proven cases of histoplasmosis have titers of only 1:8. Consequently, titers of 1:8 or higher with either antigen are considered presumptive evidence of histoplasmosis. Titer changes are of great value in diagnosing histoplasmosis. If the laboratory worker notices or suspects cross-reactions, he or she should base the diagnosis upon data derived from a study of serial serum specimens in CF and ID tests and other laboratory tests, and this should be considered in conjunction with the clinical picture.

Either the ID or the CEP test is a useful screening procedure or adjunct in the serodiagnosis of histoplasmosis. Two precipitin bands have diagnostic value (*Heiner,* 1958). One, designated "H," is rarely influenced by skin testing, and when detected, is invariably associated with active histoplasmosis. The second, designated "M," is found in acute and chronic histoplasmosis and can also appear after normal sensitized individuals have been skin-tested with histoplasmin; the demonstration of an "M" band may be indicative of active infection, inactive infection, or a recent skin test. To interpret properly the ID and CEP tests, laboratory workers must know whether the patient whose serum is being analyzed was recently histoplasmin skin-tested. If this is not so, detection of an "M" band may indicate early disease, since this band appears before the "H" band and disappears more slowly. In a recent study of sera from 52 patients with culturally proven histoplasmosis, we found that 83% were precipitin positive (*Kleger and Kaufman,* 1973). Eighty-six percent of these positive sera had "M" precipitins, 12% had both "M" and "H" precipitins and 2% had only the "H" precipitin.

The LA test provides results in 24 hours and can be used with anticomplementary sera. It is an excellent test for the diagnosis of acute histoplasmosis (*Bennett,* 1966). It may be nonreactive, however, with sera from chronically ill patients (*Campbell,* 1968). LA titers of 1:16 or greater are considered diagnostic (*Bennett,* 1966). A positive LA test should be confirmed by a CF or ID test.

Numerous investigators have shown that levels of CF antibodies, precipitins, and agglutinins to *H. capsulatum* antigens, primarily histoplasmin, may be significantly increased in histoplasmin-sensitized individuals after a single histoplasmin skin test (*Kaufman,* 1974). The antibody-inducing action of the skin test makes subsequent changes in serologic titers uninterpretable. For this reason, it is emphasized that patients with suspected histoplasmosis should not be skin tested until blood has been obtained for serological tests.

A sensitive and specific ID test (*Standard and Kaufman,* 1976) has been developed for the rapid identification of the mycelial forms of *H. capsulatum* var. *capsulatum, H. capsulatum* var. *duboisii,* and *H. farciminosum,* and for separation of these pathogenic fungi from morphologically similar hyphomycetes and other fungal pathogens. This method is based on the fact that all of the *Histoplasma spp.* produce "H" and "M" histoplasmin antigens, whereas the other fungi do not.

My experience indicates that batteries of immunologic tests are available for rapidly and accurately diagnosing many of the systemic mycotic diseases and for monitoring their course. These tests are so useful when adequately controlled and performed that they should be made an integral part of the routine diagnostic services that hospital and public health laboratories provide.

References

Bennett, D.E.: The histoplasmin latex agglutination test; clinical evaluation and a review of the literature. Am. J. med. Sci. *251:* 175–183 (1966).
Bloomfield, W.; Gordon, M.A., and Elmerdorf, D.F., jr.: Detection of *Cryptococcus neoformans* antigen in body fluid by latex particle agglutination. Proc. Soc. exp. Biol. Med. *114:* 64–67 (1963).
Bodey, G.P.: Fungal infections complicating acute leukemia. J. chron. Dis. *19:* 667–678 (1966).
Campbell, C.C.: Use and interpretation of serologic and skin tests in the respiratory mycoses: current considerations. Dis. Chest *54:* 49–54 (1968).
Coleman, R.M. and Kaufman, L.: Use of the immunodiffusion test in the serodiagnosis of aspergillosis. Appl. Microbiol. *23:* 301–309 (1972).
Goodman, J.S.; Kaufman, L., and Koenig, M.G.: Diagnosis of cryptococcal meningitis. Value of immunologic detection of cryptococcal antigen. New Engl. J. Med. *285:* 434–436 (1971).
Gordon, M.A. and Vedder, D.K.: Serologic tests in diagnosis and prognosis of cryptococcosis. J. Am. med. Ass. *197:* 961–967 (1966).
Harrell, W.K.; Ashworth, H.; Britt, L.E.; George, J.R.; Gray, S.B.; Green, J.H.; Gross, H., and Johnson, J.E.: Procedural manual for production of bacterial, fungal, and parasitic reagents (Biological Reagents Section, Center for Disease Control, Atlanta 1970).
Hart, P.D.; Russel, E., jr., and Remington, J.S.: The compromised host and infection. II. Deep fungal infection. J. infect. Dis. *120:* 169–191 (1969).
Heiner, D.C.: Diagnosis of histoplasmosis using precipitin reactions in agar gel. Pediatrics *22:* 616–627 (1958).
Huppert, M. and Bailey, J.W.: The use of immunodiffusion tests in coccidioidomycosis. Am. J. clin. Path. *44:* 364–68 (1965).
Huppert, M.; Peterson, E.T.; Sun, S.H.; Chitjian, P., and Derrevere, W.: Evaluation of a latex particle agglutination test for coccidioidomycosis. Am. J. clin. Path. *49:* 96–102 (1968).
Kaufman, L.: Serology: Its value in the diagnosis of coccidioidomycosis, cryptococcosis and histoplasmosis. Proc. Int. Symp. Mycoses Scientific Publication PAHO (No. 205), pp. 96–100 (1970).
Kaufman, L.: Serodiagnosis of fungal diseases; in Manual of clinical microbiology; 2nd ed. (Am. Soc. Microbiology, Washington 1974).
Kaufman, L. and Blumer, S.: Value and interpretation of serological tests for the diagnosis of cryptococcosis. Appl. Microbiol. *16:* 1907–1912 (1968).
Kaufman, L. and Clark, M.J.: Value of the concomitant use of complement fixation and immunodiffusion tests in the diagnosis of coccidioidomycosis. Appl. Microbiol. *28:* 641–43 (1974).
Kaufman, L.; Huppert, M.; Fava Netto, C.; Pollak, L., and Restrepo, A.: Manual of standardized serodiagnostic procedures for systematic mycoses. II. Complement fixation test. Pan Amer. Health Org., pp. 1–39 (1974).
Kaufman, L.; McLaughlin, D.W.; Clark, M.J., and Blumer, S.: Specific immunodiffusion test for blastomycosis. Appl. Microbiol. *26:* 244–247 (1973).
Kleger, B. and Kaufman, L.: Detection and identification of diagnostic *Histoplasma capsulatum* precipitates by counterelectrophoresis. Appl. Microbiol. *26:* 231–238 (1973).
Levine, H.B.; Cobb, J.M., and Scalarone, G.M.: Spherule coccidioidin in delayed dermal sensitivity reactions of experimental animals. Sabouraudia *7:* 20–32 (1969).

Pappagianis, D.; Saito, M., and Van Hoosear, K.H.: Antibody in cerebrospinal fluid in nonmenigitic coccidioidomycosis. Sabouraudia *10:* 172–179 (1972).

Parker, J.D.; Sarosi, G.A.; Doto, I.L., and Tosh, F.E.: Pulmonary aspergillosis in sanatoriums in the south central United States. Am. Rev. resp. Dis. *101:* 551–557 (1970).

Rifkind, D.; Marchioro, T.L.; Schneck, S.A., and Hill, R.B.: Systemic fungal infection complicating renal transplantation and immunosuppressive therapy. Am. J. Med. *43:* 28–38 (1967).

Schubert, J.H. and Ajello, L.: Variation in complement fixation antigenicity of different yeast phase strains of *Histoplasma capsulatum.* J. Lab. clin. Med. *50:* 304–307 (1957).

Smith, C.E.; Saito, M.T.; Beard, R.R.; Kepp, R.M.; Clark, R.W., and Eddie, B.U.: Serological tests in the diagnosis and prognosis of coccidioidomycosis. Am. J. Hyg. *52:* 1–21 (1950).

Smith, C.E.; Saito, M.T., and Simons, S.A.: Pattern of 39,500 serologic tests in coccidioidomycosis. J. Am. med. Ass. *160:* 546–552 (1956).

Stallybrass, F.C.: Candida precipitins. J. Path. Bact. *87:* 89–97 (1964).

Standard, P.G. and Kaufman, L.: A specific immunological test for the rapid identification of members of the genus *Histoplasma.* J. clin. Microbiol. *3:* 191–199 (1976).

Stickle, D.; Kaufman, L.; Blumer, S.O., and McLaughlin, D.W.: Comparison of a newly developed latex agglutination test and an immunodiffusion test in the diagnosis of systemic candidiasis. Appl. Microbiol. *23:* 490–499 (1972).

Taschdjian, C.L.; Kozinn, P.J., and Caroline, L.: Immune studies in candidiasis. III. Precipitating antibodies in systemic candidiasis. Sabouraudia *3:* 312–320 (1964).

Taschdjian, D.L.; Kozinn, P.J.; Okas, A.; Caroline, L., and Halle, M.A.: Serodiagnosis of systemic candidiasis. J. infect. Dis. *117:* 180–187 (1967).

Vogel, R.A.: The indirect fluorescent antibody test for the detection of antibody in human cryptococcal disease. J. infect. Dis. *116:* 573–580 (1966).

Wallraff, E.B.: Specific diagnostic aids in coccidioidomycosis. Clin. Med. *78:* 32–35 (1971).

Walter, J.E. and Jones, R.D.: Serologic tests in diagnosis of aspergillosis. Dis. Chest. *53:* 729–735 (1968).

Young, R.C. and Bennett, J.E.: Invasive aspergillosis – absence of detectable antibody response. Am. Rev. resp. Dis. *104:* 710–716 (1971).

Dr. *L. Kaufman,* Center for Disease Control, Public Health Service, U.S. Department of Health, Education and Welfare, *Atlanta, GA 30333* (USA)

Discussion

Dr. *Shadomy:* Would you comment upon the reliability, including both specificity and sensitivity, of commercially available serodiagnostic reagents for the mycoses.

Dr. *Kaufman:* Excellent commercial reagents are presently available for serodiagnosis of aspergillosis, blastomycosis, candidosis, coccidioidomycoses, cryptococcosis, and histoplasmosis. It is mandatory that commercial reagents or kits be checked for specificity and sensitivity with appropriate reference reagents before they are used in routine diagnostic tests. Reagents or kits producing equivocal or anomalous results should not be used, but immediately returned to the manufacturer.

Dr. *Louria:* Is it not true that it is difficult to separate colonization from invasion by *Candida* species? *Armstrong* finds that sensitivity is no more than 70% and specificity no more than 70%. How do you set up your experimental design to define sensitivity and specificity?

Dr. *Kaufman:* Yes. Patients colonized with *Candida spp.* or suffering from invasive candidosis cannot readily be distinguished by the currently used serologic procedures. The studies carried out in our laboratory indicate that the ID and LA tests for candidosis demonstrate a higher sensitivity and specificity than those noted with Dr. *Armstrong's* procedures. It is difficult to compare results since different types of patients were studied.

Sensitivity is based upon ability to react with sera from patients with proven systemic candidosis and specificity on the absence of reaction with normal sera and heterologous case sera.

Preparation of Fungal Antigens and Vaccines: Studies on *Coccidioides immitis* and *Histoplasma capsulatum*

H.B. Levine, G.M. Scalarone and S.D. Chaparas

Naval Biosciences Laboratory, University of California, School of Public Health, Berkeley, Calif., and Bureau of Biologics, Food and Drug Administration, Rockville, Md.

Antigens from *Coccidioides immitis* and *Histoplasma capsulatum* have been used extensively and successfully in clinical applications for diagnostic purposes and for prognostic indications. Preparations of sterilized culture fluid from each of these genera may be active in one or more of several immunologically mediated responses: They may react serologically in procedures that demonstrate the presence of precipitin and complement-fixing antibodies (*Smith et al.*, 1948; *Kaufman and Clark*, 1974; *Huppert et al.*, 1970; *Pappagianis et al.*, 1961; *Campbell and Saslaw*, 1948; *Scalarone et al.*, 1974); they may be cellularly-reactive *in vitro*, particularly in the mitogenic transformation of lymphocytes from sensitive donors (*Deresinski et al.*, 1974; *Chaparas et al.*, 1970); and finally, they may elicit the induration reaction of delayed sensitivity 18 to 72 hours after intracutaneous injection (*Smith et al.*, 1948; *Levine et al.*, 1973; *Stevens et al.*, 1974; *Edwards and Billing*, 1971; *Restrepo et al.*, 1968).

Considerable effort has been applied to determining qualitative and quantitative roles of coccidioidal and histoplasmal components in serologic, cellular and sensitivity reactions (*Pine*, 1957; *Campbell*, 1953; *Reeves et al.*, 1972, 1974). Fractionation procedures have led to the isolation of relatively specific antigenic moieties active in serologic reactions (*Sawaki et al.*, 1966; *Kaufman*, 1975; *Gordon*, 1975; *Pappagianis and Kobayashi*, 1958), but crude, unfractionated preparations continue to be used widely for skin testing.

Our own work has not progressed to a stage where we can point to identifiable antigens of even modest purity that are associated with one or another immunologic function. We have been concerned first with ascertaining which fungal growth forms are well-endowed with antigens of medical importance and then with procedures for obtaining the growth forms and their antigens in usable concentrations. Interest in these aspects resulted from two observations: Firstly, *C. immitis* spherule (sporangial) vaccines were strongly immunogenic, in contrast to weak immunizing activity by arthrospore and mycelial vaccines; and, secondly, coccidioidin of spherule origin elicited delayed dermal induration reactions in circumstances where sensitivity was known but where mycelial coccidioidin was nonreactive.

Spherule Vaccine

Immunological diversity among different *C. immitis* structures was demonstrated with killed vaccines in 1960 by *Levine et al.* Interest in vaccines had been stimulated by *Smith*'s observations that a coccidioidal experience in man, even if asymptomatic, was associated with the development of very strong protective immunity. In accord with his observation, experimental infections in mice produced notable resistance (*Pappagianis et al.,* 1961). Yet, formalin-killed mycelial and arthrospore vaccines were only marginally effective. Perhaps their inadequacy should have been anticipated; the arthrospore and the mycelium are saprophytic stages of the fungus. After exposure, the sojourn of the infecting arthrospore in lesions is only transitory and the occurrence of mycelia *in vivo* is infrequent. The dominant fungal structures that act as parasites in the infected host are the spherule and the endospore.

Formalin-killed vaccines, comprised of either spherules or endospores, were strikingly efficacious (*Levine et al.,* 1961, 1962, 1965). The spherule-endospore vaccine consistently protected mice against challenging doses of arthrospores more than 100-fold those lethal to non-vaccinated mice (table I). Similarly, marked protection was induced in Cynomolgous monkeys (*Levine et al.,* 1962). Credit to *J. Converse* should be given at this point because he was the first to devise a simple, chemically-defined medium that permitted the growth of spherules and endospores *in vitro;* his medium (*Converse,* 1957) made vaccine preparation possible. Only minor modification (*Levine et al.,* 1960) of the medium was necessary to adapt it to the growth of spherules of the highly immunogenic strain, Silveira, used in later studies (table I).

A well-designed experiment, demonstrating that the different immunogenic properties of spherules and mycelia were not attributable to differences in growth media or cultural conditions *per se,* was performed by *Kong and Levine* (1967). Spherules and mycelia were grown simultaneously in the same flasks of media and, after sterilization with formalin, the structures were separated and purified. Both forms were used as vaccines in mice at equal doses; the vaccinated animals were then challenged in parallel from the same arthrospore suspension. The spherule vaccine protected against a challenge of 150 LD_{50}, as compared with protection against approximately 14 LD_{50} in animals that received the mycelial vaccine.

An important consideration in the preparation of fungal vaccines was the selection of the vaccinating strain. *Huppert et al.* (1967a, b) studied the protec-

Table I. Influence of vaccination on mortality in mice infected with *Coccidioides immitis*; inter-test consistency of protective response.[1]

Naval Biosciences Laboratory Spherule-endospore vaccine Lot–J	Challenge dose (No. of arthrospores)	Dead/total control	Dead/total vaccinated
Test 1	21	3/10	nd
	36	3/10	nd
	65	6/10	0/10
	510	nd	0/10
	800	nd	0/10
Test 2	16	0/10	nd
	39	2/10	nd
	75	5/10	1/10
	630	nd	0/10
	1200	nd	0/10
Test 3	22	2/10	nd
	43	4/10	nd
	85	8/10	0/10
	626	nd	0/10
	1200	nd	1/10
Test 4	18	2/10	nd
	33	5/10	nd
	82	6/10	0/10
	555	nd	0/10
	1200	nd	0/10
Test 5	47	6/10	nd
	94	8/10	nd
	189	9/10	nd
	378	9/10	nd
	756	9/9	1/10
	1500	nd	0/10
	3030	nd	0/10
	6080	nd	0/10
	12100	nd	2/10
Test 6	50	1/10	nd
	95	6/10	0/10
	525	9/10	0/10
	2700	nd	0/10
Test 7	35	3/10	nd
	76	5/10	nd
	153	5/10	nd
	307	10/10	nd
	614	9/10	0/10
	1200	nd	0/10
	2500	nd	0/10
	4900	nd	0/10
	9800	nd	0/10

tion afforded by the strain Silveira spherule vaccine in mice challenged with arthrospores from homologous and heterologous strains. Some of the cultures had been selected for their atypical macroscopic and microscopic characteristics. Nine cultures diverse in history, origin and virulence were examined. The vaccine protected the animals in all instances; this finding led to an assumption that interstrain antigenic composition was not a major consideration with regard to a vaccination program. The validity of the assumption, it now appears, rested on the fortunate choice of strain Silveira for vaccine purposes. Other strains, examined later, yielded less effective vaccines. As an example, spherules derived from strain 46 were only very marginally protective against heterologous challenge (table II). Interestingly, despite the lack of cross-protecting immunogens in strain 46, the strain was endowed with skin-testing antigens that were effective and specific in diverse epidemiologic and clinical situations (*Levine et al.*, 1973, 1975; *Stevens et al.*, 1974, 1975).

A further determinant of immunizing efficacy in mice was related both to the morphologic phase of *C. immitis* as well as to the strain that was selected for vaccine preparation. Endospore inocula had to be employed (*Levine et al.*, 1969) to generate spherules *in vitro;* but the time for spherule maturation is strain-dependent. For optimum immunogenicity, we found that spherules had to be harvested prior to rupture, when the refractile wall was fully formed (*Levine et al.*, 1965; *Breslau*, 1957). After widespread rupture of the spherules, in the succeeding cycle of endospore release, immunogenicity diminished markedly. The spherule wall was the major locus of immunogens (*Kong et al.*, 1963). Young endospores, which may be viewed as early developing spherules, were less immunogenic than they were later; as they developed, the wall structure became more pronounced and immunogenicity increased (*Levine et al.*, 1965). Endospores harvested from mechanically-ruptured spherules were non-immunogenic. We speculate therefore that the immunogenic moieties in their walls were biosynthesized *ex utero,* or very shortly before they were released from the mother spherule.

As with bacterial vaccines, the method of killing the organism influenced the quality of the resulting product. Experience on killing agents is still limited; of eight compounds studied, formalin was the best for retaining the immunizing properties during sterilization. Cold formalin was added to chilled washed spherules in a final concentration of 0.5% and, during the 2 to 5 days required for sterilization, preparations were held at 2 to 4° C. Under similar conditions, inferior vaccines were obtained on sterilization of spherules with either ethylene

---

nd - Not done.

[1] Vaccine (0.7 mg) administered intramuscularly on days 0, 7 and 14. Animals challenged intranasally on days 41 to 53 (in different tests) and observed for a minimum of 35 additional days.

oxide, sodium hypochlorite, sodium hydroxide, benzalkonium chloride, beta propiolactone, phenol or hydrochloric acid.

The route and manner of immunization greatly influenced the protective index: Negligible immunity followed intravenous administration of the vaccine to mice. Further, the strong immunity that ordinarily was induced by intramuscular doses (tables I, II) was aborted when small amounts of vaccine were given intravenously, before immunity was evident (*Scalarone et al.,* 1971a, b; *Levine and Scalarone,* 1971). Intravenous doses, however, enhanced the response as did intramuscular doses if given when immunity was manifest. A three-fold dose regimen of 0.7 mg of spherules each, given to mice intramuscularly at intervals of one week, was life-saving under conditions of severe challenge. The response remained strong even after more than one year but was enhanced by small booster doses (*Kong et al.,* 1965).

Table II. Influence of vaccination on mortality in mice challenged with arthrospores of strains Silveira or 46[1]

Challenge doses	Dead/total (30 days after challenge) vaccinating strain		
	control	Silveira	46
Challenging strain Silveira			
25–47	9/20	nd	nd
51–94	13/20	nd	nd
100–190	14/20	nd	nd
200–380	19/20	nd	nd
400–750	18/19	1/20	1/20
900–1500	nd	0/20	6/20
1800–3000	nd	0/20	10/20
3600–6000	nd	0/20	8/20
7000–12000	nd	0/20	12/20
Challenging strain 46			
25–47	1/20	nd	nd
51–94	2/20	nd	nd
100–190	3/20	nd	nd
200–380	3/20	nd	nd
400–750	6/20	0/20	0/20
900–1500	nd	0/20	0/20
1800–3000	nd	0/20	0/20
3600–6000	nd	0/20	0/20
7000–12000	nd	0/20	3/20

[1] Summary of two experiments. Vaccinating schedule as described in table I; animals challenged intranasally on day 47 or day 53.

Spherulin

Kong et al. (1966) were the first to use a spherule-derived product to detect delayed sensitivity induced by *C. immitis*. The preparation was the supernatant fluid of spherule growth at 34° C in a casamino acid-*Converse* medium that had been stored at 4° C for 9 months. The material was termed "spherulin"; it was active at low dilution and was toxic.

Toxicity was not a problem, however, with spherulin prepared from well-washed organisms that were lysed in distilled water, rather than in their spent nutrient menstruum (*Levine et al.*, 1969; *Scalarone et al.*, 1973). Also, such preparations were active at high dilution; 10 μg were effective in sensitized mice, 5 μg elicited good reactions in infected guinea pigs (*Levine and Scalarone*, 1975) and 1.4–2.8 μg produced strong responses in human beings from *Coccidioides* endemic regions or suffering from coccidioidomycosis. The 1.4 μg spherulin dose in man produced responses comparable to those elicited by 41.6 μg of mycelium-derived coccidioidin (table III).

More important than the potency of spherulin (from strain 46) was its capacity to detect *Coccidioides*-endemic individuals from different regions who did not respond to coccidioidin. Mycelial coccidioidin is routinely prepared from a growth pool of different strains. Sixty-five cultures were represented in the reference coccidioidin of table III. The use of a multiple strain reagent was predicated on the belief that different *C. immitis* strains, possibly from different locations, had diverse antigenic profiles. The observation that spherulin detected reactors missed by coccidioidin first became apparent during epidemiological studies conducted in regions of Mexico that are endemic for coccidioidomycosis

Table III. Delayed skin sensitivity responses in five randomly selected *Coccidioides*-sensitive human volunteers tested in parallel with 1:100 coccidioidin (41.6 μg) and spherulin (1.4 μg)[1]

Test subject	Induration, mm (long and short axes)			
	24 h		48 h	
	spherulin	coccidioidin	spherulin	coccidioidin
T.J.B.	42 x 32	38 x 28	75 x 75	60 x 38
L.H.	16 x 20	14 x 11	26 x 28	22 x 20
R.B.	25 x 30	22 x 12	negative	negative
C.S.H.	28 x 40	36 x 34	46 x 52	42 x 36
J.L.R.	13 x 14	13 x 23	3 x 3	4 x 5

[1] Lot 64 $D_{2.5}$ reference coccidioidin (U.S. Food and Drug Administration, Washington, D.C.) and Lot C–104 spherulin (Berkeley Biologicals, Berkeley, California); data reproduced by kind permission of the investigator, *Thomas W. Green*, M.D., Medical Director, Berkeley Biologicals.

(*Levine et al.*, 1973). Approximately one third of spherulin-reactive individuals did not respond to coccidioidin. The finding was confirmed by other epidemiologic studies in volunteers at Livingston, California (*Stevens et al.*, 1974). Earlier, it was shown (*Levine et al.*, 1969) that spherulin elicited a sensitivity response in vaccinated mice that did not respond when tested with coccidioidin.

Stevens et al. (1975) extended the epidemiologic comparisons of spherulin and coccidioidin to the field of clinical medicine and showed the advantage of using spherulin responses in patients with clinically apparent illness or with quiescent or healed coccidioidomycosis. Of 23 patients with disseminated disease, 17 reacted with spherulin, as compared to 9 who were sensitive to coccidioidin. And among 27 patients with either disseminated disease in remission, active pulmonary disease or healed pulmonary disease, 24 were reactive with spherulin whereas 19 showed induration only with coccidioidin. Some subjects reactive with spherulin did not respond to ten times the standard dose of coccidioidin (*Steven et al.*, 1975). One patient who was anergic (unresponsive to both reagents) was treated with transfer factor from *Coccidioides*-sensitive donors; she then responded in repeated skin tests with spherulin, but not with coccidioidin. A second anergic patient, after successful treatment with Amphotericin B, acquired dermal sensitivity to spherulin before coccidioidin (*Karney and Wagner*, 1976, personal communication). Studies on lymphocyte transformation (*Deresinski et al.*, 1974) and complement fixation (*Scalarone et al.*, 1974) also indicated enhanced activity by spherulin as compared with coccidioidin. The findings as a whole were consistent with the speculation that differences between the preparations were qualitative as well as quantitative. However, as mentioned earlier, antigen fractionation studies that could establish this point definitively have not yet been done.

Despite spherulin's high sensitivity, it did not cross-react more than coccidioidin in individuals sensitized by *H. capsulatum* (*Levine et al.*, 1975). Both reagents, as well as paracoccidioidin, were compared simultaneously in 265 histoplasmin-positive Colombian soldiers from areas endemic for histoplasmosis but not for coccidioidomycosis. At standard strength, both preparations detected nonspecific responses in 0.4% (spherulin) to 1.2% (coccidioidin) of the men. At 10 times standard strength, both preparations also cross-detected histoplasmin sensitivity comparably; 5.1%–7.1% of histoplasmin-positive subjects reacted with the coccidioidal antigens. No cross-reactivity was observed between paracoccidioidin sensitivity and sensitivity to the coccidioidal antigens.

Spherulin was prepared (*Levine et al.*, 1969) by controlled lysis of washed, morphologically-purified, spherule preparations. The organisms were lysed for 40 days at $34°C$ in distilled water with shaking. Incubation periods that were shorter or longer yielded less reactive preparations (*Scalarone et al.*, 1973). Aerated incubation was superior to static incubation. Lysis at $0-4°C$ (static) produced a product that was inferior to the spherulin reagent described above.

The physical and chemical properties of the reagent as well as its storage properties have been reviewed elsewhere (*Levine and Scalarone*, 1975). Differences among preparations derived from different strains were demonstrated (*Scalarone et al.*, 1973) and the data indicated the necessity of screening strains for adequacy before selecting one for reagent preparation.

Histoplasmins –CYL and –CML

Histoplasmin has been used as a skin test antigen in epidemiological and clinical studies since 1941 when an autolysate of a dextrose broth culture of the mycelial phase of *H. capsulatum* was prepared by *Van Pernis et al.* (1941). *Emmons et al.* (1945) prepared histoplasmin for skin testing by growing the fungus in a synthetic broth medium devised for the preparation of coccidioidin. Subsequent to that time, the spent culture filtrate of mycelial growth has continued to be utilized in skin testing and serological procedures, despite the severe limitation of cross reactivity with *Blastomyces dermatitidis* and *C. immitis* or with other fungi (*Smith et al.*, 1968; *Campbell*, 1953; *Li et al.*, 1967; *Goodman*, 1971).

Numerous studies have been made on antigen preparations from *H. capsulatum* yeast cells, the cell-type characteristically present within the infected host. These included: Alcoholic precipitation of antigens from culture media (*Knight and Marcus*, 1958; *Markowitz*, 1964; *Salvin and Smith*, 1959; *Sorenson and Evans*, 1954; *Sweet*, 1971), from culture filtrates directly (*Salvin*, 1947; *Salvin and Hottle*, 1948; *Tompkins*, 1965), from disruption of yeast cells by grinding or sonication (*Campbell and Saslaw*, 1948; *Campbell*, 1953; *Pine et al.*, 1966; *Schubert and Ajello*, 1957; *Salvin and Ribi*, 1955) and complex extraction procedures (*Labzoffsky et al.*, 1957). The resulting preparations have tended to be either insensitive (*Salvin and Hottle*, 1948; *Tompkins*, 1965), unstable (*Pine et al.*, 1966), or nonspecific (*Campbell and Binkley*, 1953). Other soluble yeast phase preparations, described as specific and sensitive (*Sorenson and Evans*, 1954; *Tompkins*, 1965), have not come into general use because of the complex procedures required to isolate antigenic moieties. A relatively simple method has recently been described (*Reeves et al.*, 1972, 1974) whereby a soluble antigen was obtained from lysed yeast phase organisms in merthiolated saline. The preparation, which contained both H and M antigens as well as Y (yeast) antigen, was relatively specific, sensitive and stable in both the complement fixation and agar-gel diffusion tests. It has not been studied, however, in the skin test.

The skin-testing efficacy of spherulin, prepared by controlled lysis of spherules in water, prompted us to evaluate this methodology for the preparation of histoplasmins of yeast and mycelial origin.

The term "histoplasmin" is traditionally applied to mycelial reagents but in the present text it is used to describe either mycelial or yeast-derived prepar-

Table IV. Complete synthetic medium of *McVeigh* and *Morton* for growth of *H. capsulatum*

Component	Amount/liter
Glucose	10.0 g
KH_2PO_4	1.5 g
$MgSO_4 \cdot 7H_2O$	0.5 g
$CaCl_2 \cdot 2H_2O$	0.15 g
$(NH_4)_2SO_4$	2.0 g
L-Asparagine	2.0 g
L-Cystine[1]	0.2 g
Vitamin supplement[2]	10.0 ml
Trace element supplement[3]	1.0 ml

[1] The cystine was dissolved, prior to addition to the remainder of the medium, by heating it in a small volume of H_2O to which 1.0 N NaOH was added dropwise until solution occurred.

[2] Vitamin solution contained per 100 ml: thiamine HCl, 6.0 mg; niacin, 6.0 mg; Ca pantothenate, 6.0 mg; inositol, 1.0 g; and biotin, 0.1 mg.

[3] Trace element solution contained per 100 ml: H_3BO_3, 5.7 mg; $CuSO_4 \cdot 5H_2O$, 15.7 mg; $Fe(NH_4)_2(SO_4)_2 6H_2O$, 140.4 mg; $MnSO_4 \cdot 4H_2O$, 8.1 mg; $(NH_4)_6Mo_7O_{24} \cdot 4H_2O$, 3.6 mg; $ZnSO_4 \cdot 7H_2O$, 79.2 mg.

The components, except the vitamin supplement, were mixed and the pH adjusted to 7.0 with 1 N NaOH. After autoclaving at 121°C for 15 minutes and cooling, the filtered vitamin solution was added.

ations. "Histoplasmin-CYL" refers to a controlled yeast lysate from washed organisms in water; the term "histoplasmin-CML" describes the corresponding preparation from mycelium. In both cases, the washed organisms were lysed at 37°C with shaking as described earlier for the preparation of spherulin. In comparisons of the properties of CYL and CML reagents, the source organisms were grown as will be described, in identical defined media. However, yeasts were propagated at 37°C and mycelia at 27°C.

A vitamin-containing defined medium devised by *McVeigh and Morton* (1965) supported good growth of *H. capsulatum*. The composition is shown in table IV; yeast and mycelial skin-testing reagents derived from organisms grown in this medium gave strong reactions (medium A, fig. 1) in guinea pigs sensitized by infection. Comparable activity was obtained when the organisms were harvested from a modified medium lacking the vitamin supplement (medium C, fig. 1). The optimal duration for yeast cell lysis was 1 day (fig. 1) for the yeast reagent and 1 to 10 days for the mycelial one.

It was found that despite the comparable potency of the CYL reagents from organisms grown in media A and C, there was a medium-associated difference in specificity. Figure 2 shows that the vitamin-free medium C yielded a histoplas-

Preparation of Fungal Antigens and Vaccines

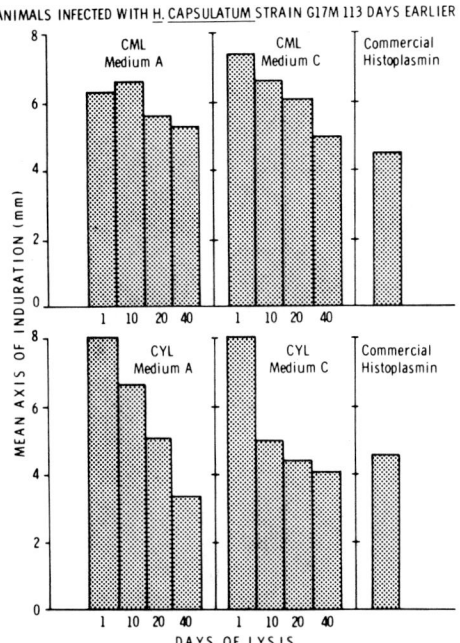

Fig. 1. Delayed sensitivity reactions of infected guinea pigs to 6 μg of histoplasmins–CML and –CYL from strain G–217A grown in the presence of vitamins (medium A) or their absence (medium C). Parke-Davis histoplasmin used at a dose of 6 μg. Ten animals per determination.

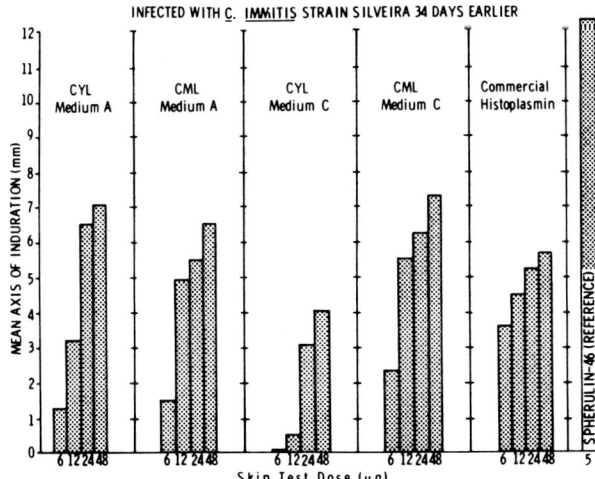

Fig. 2. Cross-reactivity (dermal) of histoplasmins–CYL and –CML in guinea pigs sensitized with *C. immitis*; influence of the presence of vitamins (medium A) or their absence (medium C). Ten animals per determination.

min-CYL reagent that did not cross react markedly in *Coccidioides*-sensitized guinea pigs unless high doses were used. Cross-reactivity was more extensive with the mycelial preparations and was not greatly altered if the preparations were derived from mycelia grown in the vitamin-deficient medium.

The influence of the source strain on the skin test activity of histoplasmins-CYL and CML was pronounced. Figure 3 shows, for example, that strain G-184A (albino) and strain G-184B (brown) yielded reagents of poor activity in guinea pigs sensitized by infection with either the homologous strain or heterologous strains, while strain G-17M, an albino strain, yielded CYL and CML reagents of higher activity. However, the maximally-reactive preparations came from strains G-217A and G-217B. All strains had been isolated from human beings with clinical histoplasmosis.

In most of the studies, CYL reagents gave stronger reactions than CML preparations. An exception, however, was observed with the CML preparation from strain G-217B (fig. 3), in both homologously- and heterologously-sensitized animals. The general superiority of the CYL reagents was demonstrated also by a different sensitization and testing scheme; table V gives the details. Guinea pigs received a high dose of killed yeast or mycelial cells in *Freund's* incomplete adjuvant. This induced strong sensitivity. The animals were then tested with the homologous strain and phase-specific reagents. In all cases the yeast preparations were more sensitive in eliciting reactions than were the mycelial preparations. As before, strain G-217A histoplasmins CYL and CML were more effective than the corresponding products from strains G-17M and

Table V. Delayed dermal sensitivity reactions in guinea pigs; responses elicited from homologous strains and morphologic phases

Sensitizing strain and growth phase[1]	Mean axis of induration[2], mm					
	G-17M		G-184A		G-217A	
	6.3 μg CML	5.6 μg CYL	20 μg CML	11 μg CYL	0.6 μg CML	0.5 μg CYL
G-17M (mycelium)	1.6					
G-17M (yeast)		8.9				
G-184A (mycelium)			4.0			
G-184A (yeast)				8.3		
G-217A (mycelium)					6.4	
G-217A (yeast)						10.0

[1] A single dose (1.3 mg-2.1 mg for different preparations) was administered subcutaneously in *Freund's* incomplete adjuvant; animals were tested 53 days later.
[2] Mean data from 4 animals per determination.

Preparation of Fungal Antigens and Vaccines 117

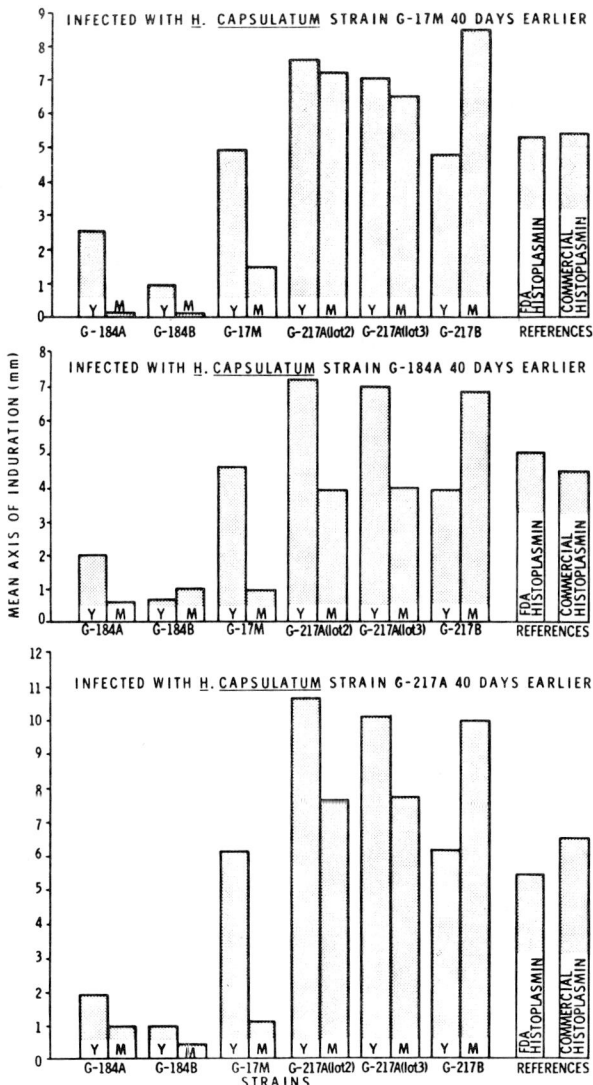

Fig. 3. Delayed dermal sensitivity reactions of infected guinea pigs to histoplasmins–CYL (Y) and –CML (M); influence of reagents from homologous and heterologous strains on reaction size. Ten animals per determination; 6 µg per dose of all reagents except the FDA reference, dose unknown, used at the recommended 1:100 dilution.

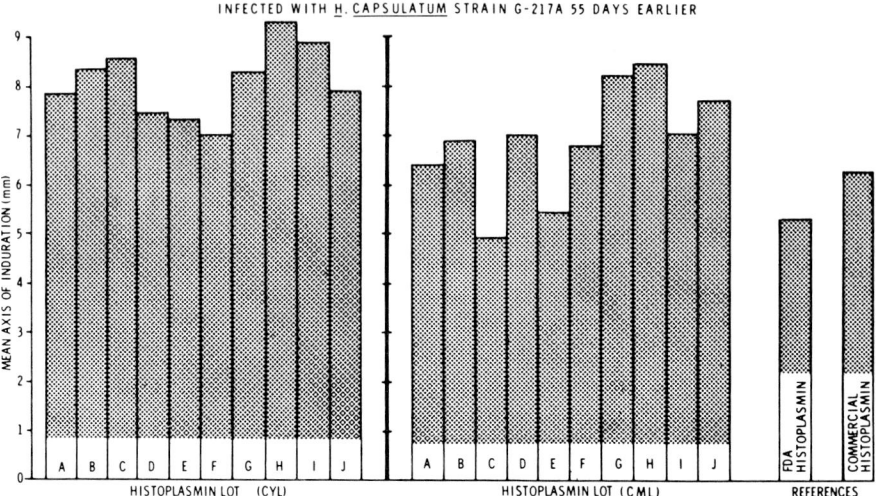

Fig. 4. Delayed dermal sensitivity reactions of infected guinea pigs to ten successive lots of histoplasmins–CYL and –CML from strain G–217A. Ten animals per determination; 6 μg per dose of all reagents except the FDA reference, dose unknown, used at the recommended 1:100 dilution.

Table VI. Delayed hypersensitivity cross-reaction (*C. immitis* infected guinea pigs) to 6 μg of CYL and CML histoplasmins prepared from *H. capsulatum* strain G–217A (10 lots each), commercial Parke-Davis histoplasmin (6 μg) and FDA reference (1:100) histoplasmin (all reactions were read "blind")

Skin test preparation	Individual guinea pig reactivity (mean axis of induration, mm)							
	1	2	3	4	5	6	7	8
G–217A–CYL Lots A–J	0	0	0	0	0	0	0	0
G–217A–CML								
Lots A, C, D, G–H	0	0	0	0	0	0	0	0
Lot B	0	0	3x3	0	0	0	0	0
Lot F	0	0	0	0	3x4	0	0	0
FDA Reference	0	3x4	3x4	0	4x4	4x5	0	3x4
Commercial histoplasmin	3x3	3x4	3x4	0	3x4	3x4	0	3x3
Spherulin–46	11x11	8x9	13x15	7x9	12x14	6x8	13x15	7x8

Table VII. Chemical properties of CYL and CML histoplasmins prepared from *H. capsulatum* strain G–217A (10 lots each)

Histoplasmins	% of total dry weight Micro-Kjeldaho (total nitrogen)	Anthrone (polysaccharide as mannose)	Folin-Ciocalteau (protein as BSA)	Protein: polysaccharide ratio
CYL				
Lot A	33	33	33	1.00
B	38	37	36	0.97
C	12	30	28	0.93
D	17	21	22	1.05
E	16	21	30	1.43
F	15	20	21	1.05
G	9	42	53	1.26
H	14	48	58	1.21
I	12	39	50	1.28
J	16	26	38	1.46
CML				
Lot A	37	18	43	2.39
B	46	9	41	4.56
C	9	8	31	3.88
D	21	23	37	1.61
E	20	27	21	0.78
F	23	49	37	0.76
G	9	55	44	0.80
H	18	44	50	1.14
I	12	53	51	0.96
J	37	47	25	0.53

G–184A. The reaction-eliciting doses for strain G–217A ranged from 0.5–0.6 µg, as compared to 5.6 µg–20 µg for the other strains.

The responses to the CYL and CML histoplasmins of strain G–217A by infected animals were examined further to determine if lot variation accounted for the superiority of the CYL preparation. Ten successive lots of CYL and CML (A–J) were prepared in parallel. Each was then tested at a dose of 6 µg, along with a commercial preparation and reference histoplasmin obtained from the Food and Drug Administration, in ten guinea pigs sensitized 55 days earlier by infection with *H. capsulatum*. A single trained individual, not one of the investigators, read the responses "blind", that is without knowing which of the 22 preparations was which. The findings are summarized in figure 4. In 8 instances, CYL produced a stronger reaction, in 1 instance the reactions were the same and in 1 case CML elicited a stronger response. In all comparisons the CYL reagents were more reactive than the corresponding dose of commercial histoplasmin and the reference standard of the Food and Drug Administration (at the recom-

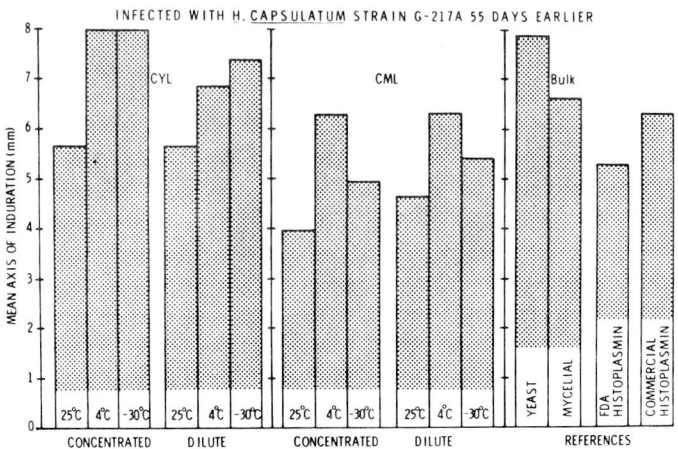

Fig. 5. Delayed dermal sensitivity reactions of infected guinea pigs to histoplasmins–CYL and –CML from strain G–217A after storage for 6 months; influence of temperature and reagent concentration (dilute at 60 μg/ml; concentrated or bulk at 290 μg/ml). Ten animals per determination; 6 μg per dose of all reagents except the FDA reference, dose unknown, used at the recommended 1:100 dilution.

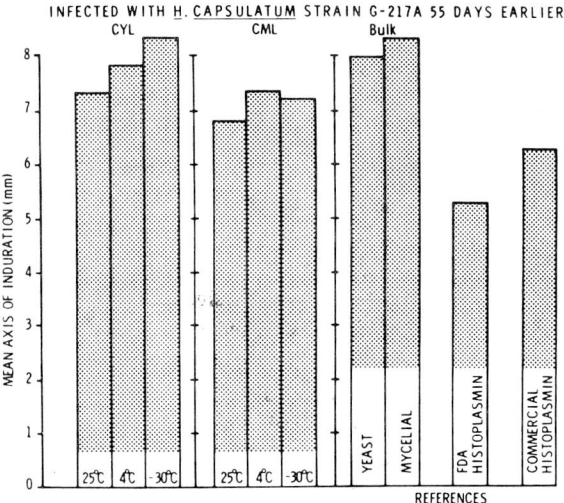

Fig. 6. Delayed dermal sensitivity reactions of infected guinea pigs to histoplasmins–CYL and –CML from strain G–217A stored lyophilized (freeze-dried) for 6 months at indicated temperatures. Ten animals per determination; 6 μg per dose of all reagents except the FDA reference, dose unknown, used at the recommended 1:100 dilution.

mended 1:100 dilution). The CML reagents were more variable (fig. 4); in two instances they were less reactive than commercial histoplasmin and in one case less than the reference preparation.

In related studies, none of the 10 CYL lots showed cross reactivity in any of 8 *Coccidioides*-sensitized guinea pigs (table VI). There were only two instances where cross-reactivity was observed in 80 responses elicited by ten CML histoplasmin lots. In contrast, 6 of the 8 *Coccidioides*-sensitive animals cross-reacted with commercial histoplasmin and 5 of these also reacted with the reference standard. All responded to spherulin.

We have found no gross chemical attributes (table VII) in specific lots of the histoplasmin reagents or in the different growth phases that could be associated with efficacy or lack of efficacy in the skin test. Probably the antigens are present in such small amounts that overall measurements of nitrogen, protein or polysaccharide are insufficient for detecting them.

The stability of the CYL and CML histoplasmins from strain G–217A is indicated in figures 5 and 6. The potency of liquid preparations diminished during six months storage at 25° C, but not very appreciably at 4° C or –30° C (fig. 5). Freeze-dried preparations, on the other hand (fig. 6), could be stored satisfactorily at 25° C or lower for at least six months.

Summary

In the past, serologic and skin testing antigens from *C. immitis* and *H. capsulatum* have often been prepared from spent culture filtrates, frequently after prolonged mycelial growth. The rationale for utilizing such a mixture reflects the observation that antigens are elaborated during growth and that different antigens may be released by autolysis at different stages of fungal development. The disadvantage of the starting material is that a multiplicity of growth byproducts will have accumulated in the mixture and desired antigens may be present only in relatively small quantities.

In our studies, three changes in the above procedure were associated with the preparation of improved antigenic reagents: (1) The tissue forms of the fungi were used (spherules in the case of *C. immitis* and yeasts in the case of *H. capsulatum*); (2) well-washed cells constituted the starting material; and (3) the antigens were obtained by controlled autolysis of the washed organisms in distilled water, not in the spent nutrient menstruum. A fourth factor influencing the quality of the preparations was the strain source for reagent preparation.

Spherulin from *C. immitis* was approximately 15–30 fold more sensitive than mycelium-derived coccidioidin in the skin test and it was also an efficacious complement-fixing antigen. Despite its increased sensitivity, it showed no more cross-reactivity in skin tests than coccidioidin in individuals sensitized by *H. capsulatum*. Yeast-derived histoplasmin has thus far been studied only in guinea pigs; it displays higher skin test sensitivity than commercial mycelial histoplasmin. At the same time, it cross-reacts less than commercial histoplasmin in animals sensitized by *C. immitis*. Both the spherulin and the histoplasmin reagents are very stable during storage at low temperature.

The immunologic influence of fungus growth phases was seen also in vaccines: Washed, formalin-killed *C. immitis* spherules (produced *in vitro*) were more immunogenic than either the arthrospore or mycelial growth phases. The immune index $\left(\frac{LD_{50} \text{ vaccinated group}}{LD_{50} \text{ control group}}\right)$ was approximately 100 for spherules compared to indices of approximately 2 to 14 for mycelia and arthrospores. Immunity was associated with heightened cellular responses, and a correlate of cellular immunity, lymphocyte transformation, was demonstrable more efficaciously with spherulin than with mycelial coccidioidin.

The data to date are in accord with the hypothesis that the tissue form of *C. immitis* possesses antigens and immunogens lacking in the mycelial form. Evidence on this point with *H. capsulatum* is less definitive; four strains in the yeast form each produced a histoplasmin reagent superior to that produced by the mycelial form but the reverse occurred with a fifth strain.

References

Breslau, A.M.: Histochemical studies on *Coccidioides immitis*. Proc. of Symp. on Coccidioidomycosis. Pub. Hlth. Serv. Pub. *575:* 189–190 (1957).

Campbell, C.C.: Antigenic fractions of *Histoplasma capsulatum*. Am. J. publ. Hlth *43:* 712–717 (1953).

Campbell, C.C. and Binkley, G.E.: Serologic diagnosis with respect to histoplasmosis, coccidioidomycosis and blastomycosis and the problem of cross reactions. J. Lab. clin. Med. *42:* 896–906 (1953).

Campbell, C.C. and Saslaw, S.: The use of yeast phase antigens in a complement fixation test for histoplasmosis. II. Results with ground antigens. J. Lab. clin. Med. *33:* 1207–1211 (1948).

Chaparas, S.D.; Sheagren J.N.; DeMeo, A., and Hedrick, S.: Correlation of skin reactivity with lymphocyte transformation induced by mycobacterial antigens and histoplasmin. Am. Rev. resp. Dis. *101:* 67–72 (1970).

Converse, J.L.: Effect of surface active agents on endosporulation of *Coccidioides immitis* in a chemically defined medium. J. Bact. *74:* 106–107 (1957).

Deresinski, S.; Levine, H.B., and Stevens, D.: Soluble antigens of mycelia and spherules in the *in vitro* detection of immunity to *Coccidioides immitis*. Infec. Immunity *10:* 700–704 (1974).

Edwards, P.Q. and Billings, E.L.: Worldwide pattern of skin sensitivity to histoplasmin. Am. J. trop. Med. Hyg. *20:* 288–319 (1971).

Emmons, C.W.; Olson, B.J., and Eldridge, W.W.: Studies in the role of fungi in pulmonary disease. I. Cross reactions of histoplasmin. Publ. Hlth Rep. *60:* 1383–1394 (1945).

Goodman, N.L.: Cross reactivity in histoplasmin skin testing; in *Ajello, Chick and Furcolow* Histoplasmosis (Thomas, Springfield 1971).

Gordon, M.: Current status of serology for diagnosis and prognostic evaluation of opportunistic fungus infections. Proc. 3rd. Int. Conf. on the Mycoses, Sci. Publ. *304:* 144–153 (Pan American Health Organization, Washington 1975).

Huppert, M.; Chitjian, P.A., and Gross, A.J.: Comparison of methods for coccidioidomycosis complement fixation. Appl. Microbiol. *20:* 328–332 (1970).

Huppert, M.; Levine, H.B.; Sun, S.H., and Peterson, E.T.: Resistance of vaccinated mice to typical and atypical strains of *Coccidioides immitis*. J. Bact. *94:* 924–927 (1967a).

Huppert, M.; Sun, S.H., and Bailey, J.: Natural variability in *Coccidioides immitis*. Proc. 2nd Coccidioidomycosis Symp., Tucson, 1965 (University of Arizona Press, Tucson 1967b).

Kaufman, L.: Current status of immunology for diagnosis and prognostic evaluation of blastomycosis, coccidioidomycosis and paracoccidioidomycosis. Proc. 3rd Int. Conf. on the Mycoses., Sci. Publ. *304:* 137–143 (Pan American Health Organization, Washington 1975).

Kaufman, L. and Clark, M.J.: Value of the concomitant use of complement fixation and immunodiffusion tests in the diagnosis of coccidioidomycosis. Appl. Microbiol. *28:* 641–643 (1974).

Knight, R.A. and Marcus, S.: Polysaccharide skin-test antigens derived from *Histoplasma capsulatum* and *Blastomyces dermatitidis.* Am. Rev. Tuberc. *77:* 983–989 (1958).

Kong, Y.M. and Levine, H.B.: Experimentally induced immunity in the mycoses. Bact. Rev. *31:* 35–53 (1967).

Kong, Y.M.; Savage, D.C., and Levine, H.B.: Enhancement of immune responses in mice by a booster injection of coccidioidal spherules. J. Immun. *95:* 1048–1056 (1965).

Kong, Y.M.; Savage, D.C., and Kong, N.L.: Delayed dermal hypersensitivity in mice to spherule and mycelial extracts of *Coccidioides immits.* J. Bact. *91:* 876–883 (1966).

Kong, Yi-chi, M.; Levine, H.B., and Smith, C.E.: Immunogenic properties of nondisrupted and disrupted spherules of *Coccidioides immitis.* in mice. Sabouraudia *2:* 131–142 (1963).

Labzoffsky, N.A.; Fischer, J.B., and Hamvas, J.J.: Studies on the antigenic structure of *Histoplasma capsulatum.* Can. J. Microbiol. *3:* 975–985 (1957).

Levine, H.B. and Scalarone, G.M.: Deficient resistance to *Coccidioides immitis* following intravenous vaccination. III. Humoral and cellular responses to intravenous and intramuscular doses. Sabouraudia *9:* 97–108 (1971).

Levine, H.B. and Scalarone, G.M.: Properties of spherulin, a skin test reagent in coccidioidomycosis. Proc. 3rd Int. Conf. on the Mycoses, Sci. Publ. *304:* 101–110 (Pan American Health Organization, Washington 1975).

Levine, H.B.; Cobb, J.M., and Scalarone, G.M.: Spherule coccidioidin in delayed dermal sensitivity reactions of experimental animals. Sabouraudia *7:* 20–32 (1969).

Levine, H.B.; Cobb, J.M., and Smith, C.E.: Immunity to coccidioidomycosis induced in mice by purified spherule, arthrospore and mycelial vaccines. Trans. N.Y. Acad. Sci. *22:* 436–449 (1960).

Levine, H.B.; Cobb, J.M., and Smith, C.E.: Immunogenicity of spherule-endospore vaccines of *Coccidioides immitis* for mice. J. Immun. *87:* 218–227 (1961).

Levine, H.B.; Gonzalez Ochoa, A., and Ten Eyck, D.R.: Dermal sensitivity to *Coccidioides immitis.* A comparison of responses elicited in man by spherulin and coccidioidin. Am. Rev. resp. Dis. *107:* 379–386 (1973).

Levine, H.B.; Kong, Y.M.; and Smith, C.E.: Immunization of mice to *Coccidioides immitis.* Dose, regimen and spherulation stage of killed spherule vaccines. J. Immun. *94:* 132–142 (1965).

Levine, H.B.; Miller, R.L., and Smith, C.E.: Influence of vaccination on respiratory coccidioidal disease in Cynomologous monkeys. J. Immun. *89:* 242–251 (1962).

Levine, H.B.; Restrepo, M.A.; Ten Eyck, D.R., and Stevens, D.A.: Spherulin and coccidioidin: Cross-reactions in dermal sensitivity to histoplasmin and paracoccidioidin. Am. J. Epidem. *101:* 512–516 (1975).

Li, M.; Garrison, R.G., and Dodd, H.: Complement fixing cross reactivity between *Histoplasma capsulatum* and certain form-related aleuriosporic hyphomycetes. Mycopath. Mycol. appl. *33:* 353–363 (1967).

Markowitz, H.: Polysaccharide skin test antigens from *Histoplasma capsulatum.* Proc. Soc. exp. Biol. Med. *115:* 697–700 (1964).

McVeigh, I. and Morton, K.: Nutritional studies of *Histoplasma capsulatum.* Mycopath. Mycol. appl. *25:* 294–308 (1965).

Pappagianis, D. and Kobayashi, G.S.: Production of extracellular polysaccharide in cultures of *Coccidioides immitis.* Mycologia *50:* 229–238 (1958).

Pappagianis, D.; Levine, H.B.; Smith, C.E.; Berman, R.J., and Kobayashi, G.S.: Immunization of mice with viable *Coccidioides immitis.* J. Immun. *86:* 28–34 (1961).

Pappagianis, D.; Smith, C.E.; Kobayashi, G.S., and Saito, M.T.: Studies on antigens from young mycelia of *Coccidioides immitis.* J. infect. Dis. *108:* 35 (1961).

Pine, L.: Studies on the growth of *Histoplasma capsulatum.* III. Effect of thiamin and other vitamins on the growth of yeast and mycelial phase of *Histoplasma capsulatum.* J. Bact. *74:* 239–245 (1957).

Pine, L.; Boone, C.J., and McLaughlin, D.: Antigenic properties of the cell wall and other fractions of the yeast form of *Histoplasma capsulatum.* J. Bact. *91:* 2158–2168 (1966).

Reeves, M.W.; Pine, L., and Bradley, G.: Characterization and evaluation of a soluble antigen complex prepared from the yeast phase of *Histoplasma capsulatum.* Infec. Immunity *9:* 1033–1044 (1974).

Reeves, M.W.; Pine, L.; Kaufman, L., and McLaughlin, D.: Isolation of a new soluble antigen from the yeast phase of *Histoplasma capsulatum.* Appl. Microbiol. *24:* 841–843 (1972).

Restrepo, A.M.; Robledo, M.V.; Ospina, S.C.; Restrepo, M.I. and Correa, A.L.: Distribution of paracoccidioidin sensitivity in Colombia. Am. J. trop. Med. Hyg. *17:* 25–37 (1968).

Salvin, S.B.: Complement-fixation studies in experimental histoplasmosis. Proc. Soc. exp. Biol. Med. *66:* 324–325 (1947).

Salvin, S.B. and Hottle, G.A.: Serologic studies on antigens from *Histoplasma capsulatum* Darling. J. Immun. *60:* 57–66 (1948).

Sawaki, Y.; Huppert, M.; Bailey, J.W., and Yagi, Y.: Patterns of human antibody reactions in coccidioidomycosis. J. Bact. *91:* 422–427 (1966).

Salvin, S.B. and Ribi, E.: Antigens from yeast phase of *Histoplasma capsulatum.* II. Immunologic properties of protoplasm vs. cell walls. Proc. Soc. exp. Biol. Med. *90:* 287–294 (1955).

Salvin, S.B. and Smith, R.F.: Antigens from the yeast phase of *Histoplasma capsulatum.* III. Isolation, properties, and activity of a protein-carbohydrate complex. J. infect. Dis. *105:* 45–53 (1959).

Scalarone, G.M. and Levine, H.B.: Deficient resistance to *Coccidioides immitis* following intravenous vaccination. I. Distribution of spherules after intravenous and intramuscular doses. Sabouraudia *9:* 81–89 (1971a).

Scalarone, G.M. and Levine, H.B.: Deficient resistance to *Coccidioides immitis* following intravenous vaccination. II. Evidence against an immune tolerance mechanism. Sabouraudia *9:* 90–96 (1971b).

Scalarone, G.M.; Levine, H.B.; Chaparas, S.D., and Cobb, J.M.: Properties and assay of spherulins from *Coccidioides immitis* in delayed sensitivity responses of animals. Sabouraudia *11:* 222–234 (1973).

Scalarone, G.M.; Levine, H.B.; Pappagianis, D., and Chaparas, S.D.: Spherulin as a complement fixing antigen in human coccidioidomycosis. Am. Rev. resp. Dis. *110:* 324–328 (1974).

Schubert, J.H. and Ajello, L.: Variation in complement fixation antigenicity of different yeast phase strains of *Histoplasma capsulatum.* J. Lab. clin. Med. *50:* 304–307 (1957).

Smith, C.E.; Whiting, E.G.; Baker, E.E.; Rosenberger, H.G.; Beard, R.R., and Saito, M.T.: The use of coccidioidin. Am. Rev. Tuberc. Pulm. Dis. *57:* 330–360 (1948).

Sorenson, L.J. and Evans, E.E.: Antigenic fractions specific for *Histoplasma capsulatum* in the complement-fixation reaction. Proc. Soc. exp. Biol. Med. *87:* 339–341 (1954).

Stevens, D.A.; Levine, H.B.; Deresinski, S., and Blaine, L.J.: Spherulin in clinical coccidioidomycosis. Chest *68:* 697–702 (1975).

Stevens, D.A.; Levine, H.B., and Ten Eyck, D.R.: Dermal sensitivity to different doses of spherulin and coccidioidin. Chest. *65:* 530–533 (1974).

Sweet, G.H.: Antigens of *Histoplasma capsulatum.* II. Separation and characterization of yeast phase precipitinogens. Am. Rev. resp. Dis. *104:* 401–407 (1971).

Tompkins, V.N.: Soluble antigenic constituents of yeast phase *Histoplasma capsulatum.* Am. Rev. resp. Dis. *92:* suppl., pp. 126–133 (1965).

Van Pernis, P.A.; Benson, M.E., and Holinger, P.H.: Specific cutaneous reactions with histoplasmosis. J. Am. med. Ass. *117:* 436–437 (1941).

Dr. *H.B. Levine,* Naval Biosciences Laboratory, University of California, School of Public Health, *Berkeley, CA 94720* (USA)

Contr. Microbiol. Immunol., vol. 3, pp. 126–137 (Karger, Basel 1977)

Antigenic Relationships of *Candida albicans, Saccharomyces telluris* and *Saccharomyces cerevisiae*

H.F. Hasenclever and F.J. McAtee

U.S. Department of Health, Education, and Welfare, Public Health Service, National Institutes of Health, National Institute of Allergy and Infectious Diseases, Rocky Mountain Laboratory, Hamilton, Mont.

A recent report (*Hasenclever and Kocan,* 1973) indicated the presence of serotypes within the species of yeast *Saccharomyces telluris*. Because of our interest in antigens of yeasts, we have studied the serologic cross reactivity among the two antigenic groups of *Candida albicans* and the three serotyes of *S. telluris*. A considerable amount of knowledge is available concerning the structural (*Yu et al.,* 1967) and the serological properties of the antigenic groups of *C. albicans* (*Hasenclever and Mitchell,* 1964; *Summers et al.,* 1964; *Sunayama,* 1970; *Sunayama and Suzuki,* 1970). Therefore, comparison of the serologic reactivity of the *S. telluris* serotypes with that of the antigenic groups of *C. albicans* should yield useful information concerning the chemical composition and structure of the antigens of the former. *S. cerevisiae* was included in this study because of the knowledge contributed by the work of *Suzuki et al.* (1968) and *Ballou* (1974) defining the haptenic groups for the mannan of this yeast and the work of *Ballou* (1974) describing biosynthetic pathways for mannan formation. The results presented here were obtained employing quantitative precipitin reactions using mannans or polysaccharides extracted from yeast cells.

Methods

Strains of yeasts. *C. albicans* 311A and 792B, two strains that have been used extensively by ourselves and others in studying the antigenic characteristics of this species, were used. *S. telluris* 2676, Serotype A, and 2685, Serotype C, were obtained from the Centraalbureau voor Schimmelcultures, Delft, Netherlands. *S. telluris* 3197, Serotype B, was isolated from *Columba livia,* the common pigeon. *S. cerevisiae* was a strain of brewer's yeast.

[1] We gratefully acknowledge the contribution of *William Bickel* in performing the phosphorus and nitrogen determinations on the polysaccharides.

Antisera. Antisera were raised by injecting rabbits intravenously with suspensions containing 10^9 heat-killed yeast cells per ml. 1 ml injections were given daily or four times a week to a total of 12–14 injections. All antisera demonstrated an agglutinin titer of 1:640 or more and all those antisera raised by the antigenically more complex strains showed their typical group or serotypic specificity after absorption with the appropriate yeast cells. Sera were absorbed following a procedure previously described (*Hasenclever and Mitchell,* 1960).

Antigens. Yeast cells. The yeast cells used for immunization, absorption, and extraction of polysaccharides were harvested from 0.5% yeast extract, 2% glucose, 1% neopeptone broth cultures grown at 37° C for 1–2 days. The cells were washed three times with sterile distilled H_2O; viability in those cells used for immunization and absorption was destroyed by autoclaving for 15 minutes at 121° C. The cells were then washed and suspended in 0.85% NaCl solution. Cell concentrations were determined using a Klett-Summerson photoelectric colorimeter.

Polysaccharides were extracted from whole yeast cells using the method of *Peat et al.* (1961). This procedure is particularly effective in the isolation and purification of mannans. In brief, 50% cell suspensions in $0.02M$ Na citrate solution were autoclaved for three hours at 121° C, then centrifuged and the supernatant fluid poured off and retained. Another volume of Na citrate was added, the cells were resuspended, autoclaved another three hours, centrifuged, and the supernate was then pooled with the first. Fehling's solution was added to the pooled supernates and the polysaccharide precipitated as a Cu complex. The precipitate was dissolved in H_2O, acidified, the Cu ions removed with the ion exchange resin Dowex #50, and the polysaccharide precipitated with ethanol. The precipitate was redissolved in H_2O and the alcoholic precipitation process repeated two or three times. The final precipitate was again redissolved in H_2O and freeze-dried. The resultant extract was a white, fluffy, amorphous material, soluble in H_2O at 8 mg or more per ml. Analyses of the polysaccharides used in this study for total sugar (*Dubois et al.,* 1956), nitrogen (*Johnson,* 1941), and phosphorus (*Dryer et al.,* 1957) are shown in table I. Earlier studies on the polysaccharides isolated from the two strains of *C. albicans* and *S. cerevisiae* by this method of extraction indicated that they were 95% mannose and 5% glucose (*Hasenclever and Mitchell,* 1964; *Summers et al.,* 1964). The monosaccharide(s) of the polysaccharides extracted from the serotypes of *S. telluris* were not identified chemically. Their serologic cross reactivity with *C. albicans* and *S. cerevisiae* antisera suggests that mannose is a major component.

Serological procedures. Quantitative precipitation. The method described by *Gitlin* (1949) for calculating antibody protein in immune precipitates was used. For this investigation, 0.1 ml of antiserum was placed in each tube and five to seven antigen concentrations were utilized, the number depending upon the amount of antigen required to achieve maximum precipitation. All tests were done in duplicate and the data averaged to calculate

Table I. Composition of polysaccharides

		% nitrogen	% phosphorus	% sugar
S.t.	A 2676	1.97	0.27	90
S.t.	B 3197	2.63	0.49	89
S.t.	C 2685	2.72	0.34	88
C.a.	A 311	0.34	0.25	96
C.a.	B 792	0.16	0.86	98
S.c.		0.96	<0.1	96

the final value of antibody precipitated. The antigen-antiserum mixtures were thoroughly shaken and placed in a water-bath at 37° C for 1½–2 hours. After incubation, they were maintained at 4° C for 2 to 3 days. The precipitates were then washed three times in 0.15 M phosphate-buffered saline and dissolved in 0.25 N acetic acid. The protein concentration of the dissolved precipitates was determined by absorbance measurements at 277 nm in a Beckman model DU spectrophotometer. The protein that was present in the precipitate was considered to be antibody protein. Although nitrogen was present in varying amounts in the antigens used in these tests, corrections for nitrogen content were not made, for reasons stated below.

Immunodiffusion using these polysaccharides has been tried but the results have been so variable and difficult to interpret that they are not included in this report.

Results and Discussion

The chemical analyses of the mannans isolated from the two *C. albicans* strains and *S. cerevisiae* and the polysaccharides extracted from the three serotypes of *S. telluris* are shown in table I. If nitrogen content is used as the basis for impurity, it appears that the mannans of *C. albicans* A and B are the most pure, *S. cerevisiae* next, and the polysaccharides from the serotypes of *S. telluris* the least pure. The lower sugar content of the *S. telluris* polysaccharides is probably due to their higher nitrogen content.

The phosphorus content, which varied, was probably in the form of phosphate diesters (*Stewart and Ballou*, 1969). The high level in *C. albicans* 792 and the trace amounts in *S. cerevisiae* have been reported by other investigators.

Quantitative precipitin reactions of the various polysaccharides with unabsorbed antiserum to *S. telluris* A are shown in figure 1. It is apparent that the amount of antibody precipitated by *C. albicans* A and *S. telluris* A is quite similar. Precipitation by the other polysaccharides was much less.

The precipitin curves for *S. telluris* B antiserum are shown in figure 2. The homologous reaction was the strongest and *S. telluris* A was next, precipitating about two-thirds as much antibody protein. The polysaccharides of *C. albicans* A and *S. telluris* C were quite similar in their reactivity.

The results with antiserum to *S. telluris* C are shown in figure 3. The homologous reaction was the strongest with *S. telluris* B, and A was next in precipitating activity.

Figure 4 shows the precipitating activity for the polysaccharides with *C. albicans* A antiserum. The homologous reaction and that with *S. telluris* A are practically identical. It appears from the results shown in this figure and in figure 1 that the haptenic groups of the polysaccharides from *C. albicans* A and *S. telluris* A are very similar. All the other heterologous polysaccharides show considerable reactivity with this antiserum.

The reactions with antiserum to *C. albicans* B are shown in figure 5. The heterologous reaction with *C. albicans* A mannan is stronger than the homol-

Antigenic Relationships of *Candida albicans*

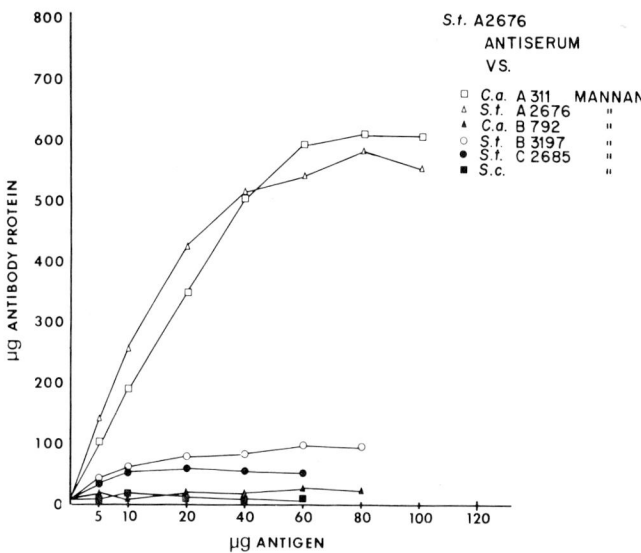

Fig. 1. Precipitin reactions with unabsorbed antiserum to *S. telluris* A.

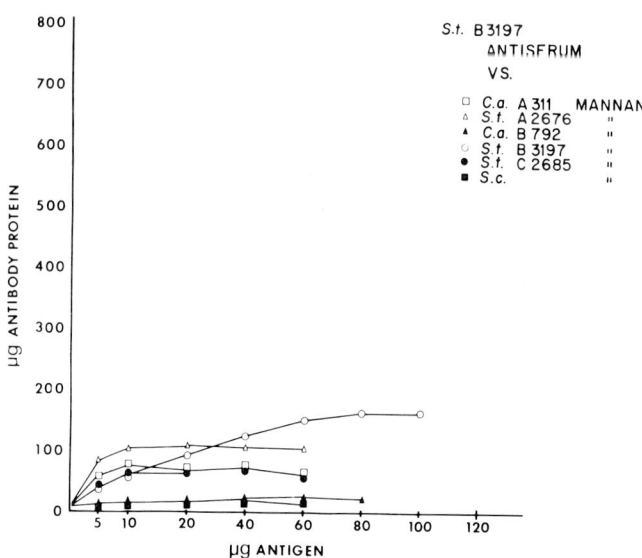

Fig. 2. Precipitin reactions with unabsorbed antiserum to *S. telluris* B.

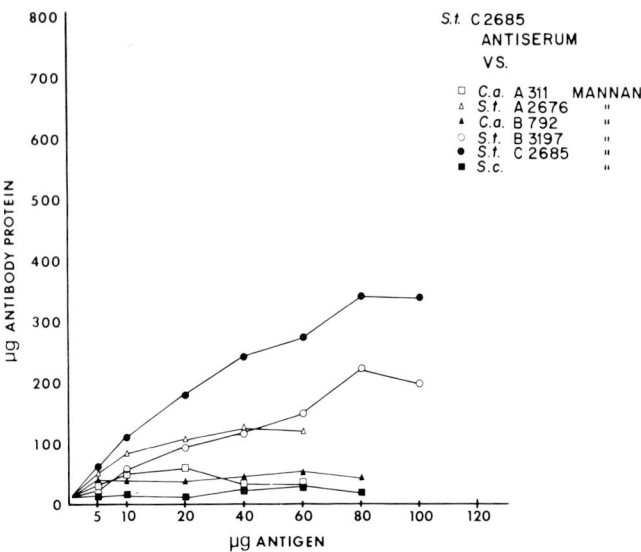

Fig. 3. Precipitin reactions with unabsorbed antiserum to *S. telluris* C.

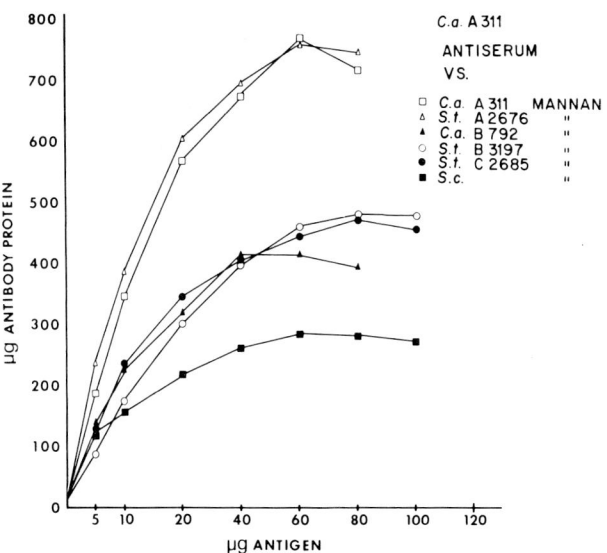

Fig. 4. Precipitin reactions with unabsorbed antiserum to *C. albicans* A.

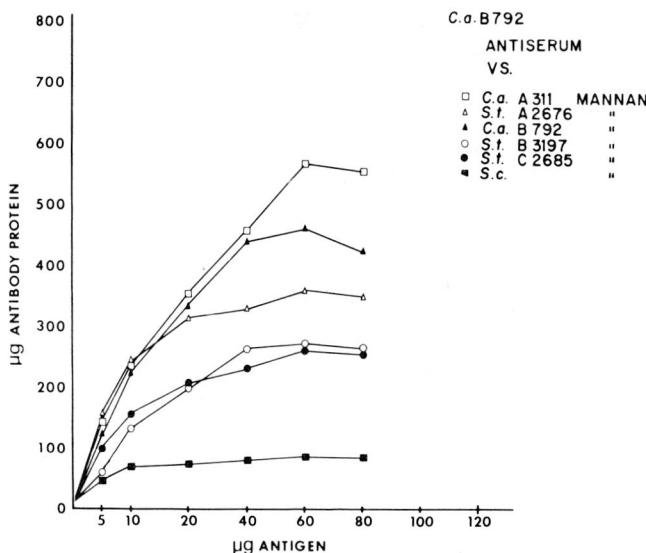

Fig. 5. Precipitin reactions with unabsorbed antiserum to *C. albicans* B.

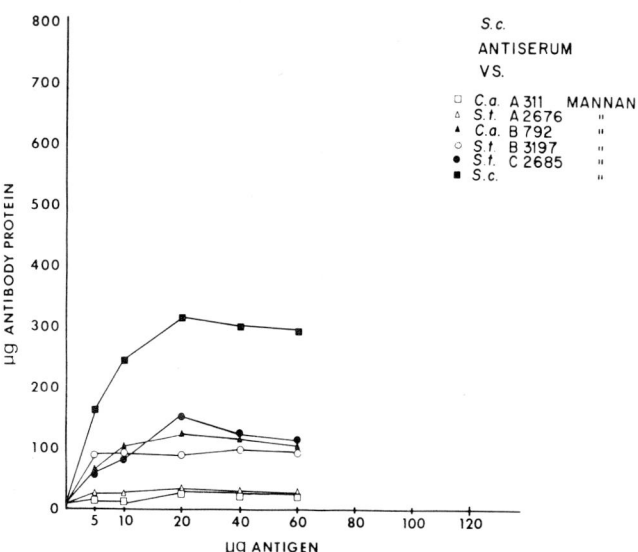

Fig. 6. Precipitin reactions with unabsorbed antiserum to *S. cerevisiae*.

ogous reaction. Although this phenomenon has been noted before (*Hasenclever and Mitchell,* 1964) we have no explanation for it. The polysaccharides from the serotypes of *S. telluris* were considerably more reactive in precipitating this antiserum than *C. albicans* B mannan was in precipitating antisera to the serotypes.

The results with antiserum to *S. cerevisiae* are shown in figure 6. The homologous mannan precipitated about twice as much antibody as the next closest polysaccharide. Mannan of *S. cerevisiae* precipitated approximately 30% of the *C. albicans* A antibody (fig. 4) but *C. albicans* A mannan precipitated no more than 10% of the *S. cerevisiae* antibody. The polysaccharides of *S. telluris* B and C and *C. albicans* B were more reactive in precipitating *S. cerevisiae* antiserum than the mannan of *S. cerevisiae* was in precipitating antisera to these yeasts.

No correction for the possible contribution of the nitrogen content in the polysaccharide to the total protein in the immune precipitate was made. If it is assumed that all of the nitrogen was precipitated in the immune complex, even with *S. telluris* (fig. 2) at 100 μg of antigen, the correction (16.4 μg) for the homologous reaction (165 μg antibody protein) would have been 10%. The correction for the *S. telluris* C homologous reaction (345 μg antibody protein) would have been approximately 5%. For some of the heterologous reactions where maximal precipitation occurred with 10–20 μg (*S. telluris* B antiserum) the corrective factor would have been negligible. Even where a correction of 10% could have been made, interpretations of the results would not have been affected. The need for a correction is based upon the assumption that all of the antigen nitrogen was serologically active or bound to serologically active polysaccharides and thus precipitated in the immune complex. There is no information to either support or contradict this assumption.

Since absorbed sera were necessary to show qualitative differences among the serotypes of *S. telluris* (*Hasenclever and Kocan,* 1973) and groups of *C. albicans* (*Summers et al.,* 1964) by agglutination, they were also used to determine if serologic similarities or dissimilarities could be demonstrated in the polysaccharides extracted from the yeasts under study. Only those absorbed antisera that were considered might provide useful information, based upon results obtained with the unabsorbed antisera, were selected.

Antiserum to *S. telluris* A absorbed with cells of *C. albicans* A was not precipitated by any of the polysaccharides. This illustrates the close antigenic relationship between *S. telluris* A and *C. albicans* A.

Precipitation by the polysaccharides from *S. telluris* A and *C. albicans* A with antiserum to *S. telluris* A absorbed with *S. telluris* B cells is shown in figure 7 (bottom). Both extracts were quite reactive. Since *C. albicans* B mannan only very slightly precipitated the unabsorbed *S. telluris* A antiserum, it was not tested.

Data for antiserum to *S. telluris* A absorbed with *S. telluris* C cells are shown in figure 7 (middle). Precipitation by the *S. telluris* A polysaccharides and

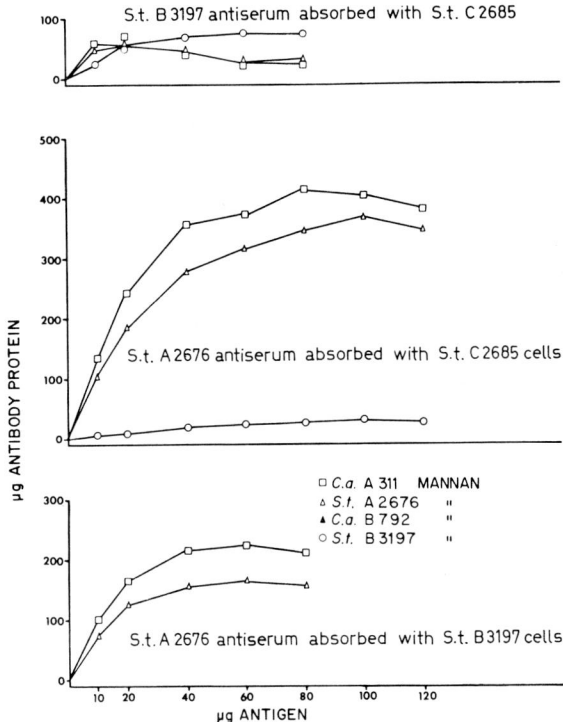

Fig. 7. Bottom: Precipitation by the polysaccharides of *S. telluris* A and *C. albicans* A with antiserum to *S. telluris* A absorbed with the cells of *S. telluris* B. *Middle:* Precipitation by the polysaccharides of *S. telluris* A, B, and *C. albicans* A with antiserum to *S. telluris* A absorbed with the cells of *S. telluris* C. *Top:* Precipitation by the polysaccharides of *S. telluris* A, B, and *C. albicans* A with antiserum to *S. telluris* B absorbed with the cells of *S. telluris* C.

the *C. albicans* A mannan can be noted. The reaction with the *S. telluris* B polysaccharide was quite slight, but detectable.

The reactivity of the polysaccharides extracted from *S. telluris* A and B and the mannan of *C. albicans* A with antiserum to *S. telluris* B absorbed with *S. telluris* C cells is shown in figure 7 (top). All three polysaccharides precipitated the antiserum. Because *C. albicans* B mannan was quite unreactive with the unabsorbed antiserum, it was not tested.

Data for *C. albicans* A antiserum absorbed with *S. telluris* A cells are shown in figure 8 (bottom). Although antibody protein could be detected, the values were at the minimum of the sensitivity of the method and differences can only be regarded as qualitative.

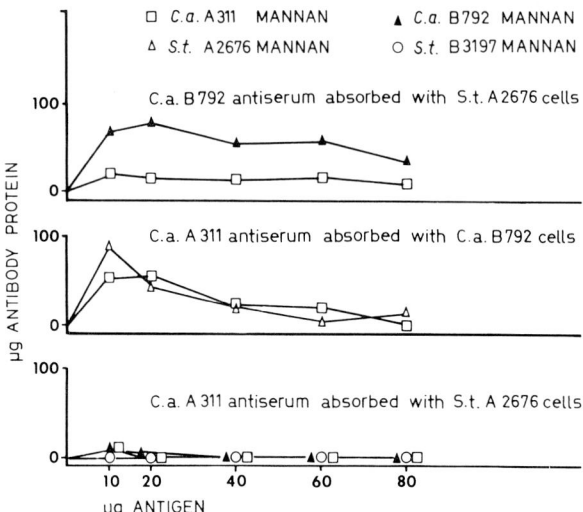

Fig. 8. Bottom: Precipitation by the mannans of *C. albicans* A and B with antiserum to *C. albicans* A absorbed with the cells of *S. telluris* A. *Middle:* Precipitation by the polysaccharides of *S. telluris* A and *C. albicans* A with antiserum to *C. albicans* A absorbed with the cells of *C. albicans* B. *Top:* Precipitation by the mannans of *C. albicans* A and B with antiserum to *C. albicans* B absorbed with the cells of *S. telluris* A.

Precipitation of *C. albicans* A antiserum absorbed with the cells of *C. albicans* B by *C. albicans* A mannan and *S. telluris* polysaccharide is shown in figure 8 (middle). The curves indicate that the A specificity was present in both polysaccharides.

The reactions of *C. albicans* A and B mannans with *C. albicans* B antiserum absorbed with *S. telluris* A cells are shown in figure 8 (top). Both mannans were reactive but the homologous precipitation was stronger. This suggests that the *C. albicans* B mannan possesses some determinants that are not present on the *C. albicans* A mannan; this was not noted in an earlier study (*Summers et al.*, 1964) when *C. albicans* B antiserum was absorbed with *C. albicans* A cells. *Sunayama* (1970), absorbing *C. albicans* B antiserum with mannan from *C. albicans* A, also did not find any haptenic determinants on the B mannan that were not present on the A mannan.

The quantitative antigenic similarities between *C. albicans* A and *S. telluris* A as shown by precipitation are apparent. The close serologic relationship between the *S. telluris* A polysaccharide and the *C. albicans* A mannan suggests strongly that the former is also a mannan, with a structure quite similar to that of the *C. albicans* A mannan. *Sunayama* (1970) has shown, by precipitin inhibition, that $\alpha 1 \rightarrow 2$ linked mannohexaose and mannoheptaose moieties constitute the Group A specificity. Further studies by *Sunayama and Suzuki* (1970) have demonstrated that the principal haptenic determinants of *C. albicans* B mannan are α 1 → 2 linked mannopentaose and mannotetraose units and that *C. albicans* A mannan also possesses these determinants, which for both mannans are branches joined to an α 1 → 6 linked mannose core or backbone. Although the branches are predominantly of the α 1 → 2 configuration, a few α 1 → 3 linkages are known to be present. *C. albicans* A antiserum absorbed with *C. albicans* B is precipitated by the *C. albicans* A mannan and the polysaccharide of *S. telluris* A; therefore this latter must contain some mannohexaose or mannoheptaose determinants. Conversely, since *C. albicans* B antiserum absorbed with *S. telluris* A is precipitated by either *C. albicans* mannan, *S. telluris* A must not possess all of the antigenic determinants of the *C. albicans* mannans. The low reactivity of the *C. albicans* B mannan with unabsorbed antiserum to *S. telluris* A suggests that this mannan possesses relatively few determinants that are common to this serotype. From the knowledge available, we would predict that the *S. telluris* A polysaccharide lacks some of the determinants that are composed of fewer mannose units.

Less can be said about the structures of the polysaccharides from *S. telluris* B and C except to suggest, from their precipitation of the antisera to *C. albicans* A, B and *S. cerevisiae,* that they are composed mostly of mannose.

Suzuki et al. (1968) have shown that the principal antigenic determinants of the mannan of *S. cerevisiae* were branches with an α 1 → 2 linked mannotetraose unit containing a terminal α 1 → 3 linkage, and an α 1 → 2 linked mannotriose oligosaccharide. With the exception of *C. albicans* A antiserum, *S. cerevisiae* mannan was quite unreactive with heterologous antisera. It would appear therefore that these unreactive heterologous antisera did not possess combining sites reactive with the *S. cerevisiae* determinants. On the other hand, the polysaccharides of *S. telluris* B, C and *C. albicans* B precipitated about 30% of the *S. cerevisiae* antibody but *C. albicans* A mannan no more than 10%. This lack of cross reactive reciprocity is puzzling but may be due to spatial arrangements of the determinants or branches on the mannan core which in some instances results in interference with antibody combination.

In general, the antigenic relationships of the serotypes of *S. telluris* (*Hasenclever and Kocan,* 1973) shown to be present on the yeast cells could also be demonstrated in polysaccharides extracted from the yeast cells. It cannot be denied that during the extraction procedure some antigenic properties may have been destroyed. It is known from studies on *S. cerevisiae* that the mannan of the yeast cell surface exists as a mannan-protein complex (*Ballou,* 1974). The role of this surface protein as an antigen remains unknown. Antisera of *C. albicans* raised in sheep or rabbits by immunizing with whole yeast cells or mannans, extracted by this same procedure and mixed in complete *Freund*'s adjuvant, showed no differences in their reactivity (*Hasenclever and Mitchell,* 1964).

More work remains to be done before all the antigenic relationships among these yeasts are known. All absorptions of antisera were carried out using whole yeast cells and we have not absorbed antisera using mannans or polysaccharides. Animals have not been immunized with the polysaccharides from the serotypes of *S. telluris* and the antisera compared with those raised by whole cells. The qualitative monosaccharide content of the *S. telluris* polysaccharides needs to be determined and their structure studied. With a better knowledge of the surface antigens of yeasts and their immunogenicity, the reasons for their cross reactivity can be characterized and utilized for possible taxonomic applications and for a better understanding of the immune response to yeast infections.

Summary

A close antigenic relationship between *C. albicans* A and *S. telluris* A was found. The serologic differences among the serotypes of *S. telluris* were noted in the extractable polysaccharides. Cross reactions with absorbed and unabsorbed antisera to *C. albicans* A and B and unabsorbed antiserum to *S. cerevisiae* suggested that these polysaccharides were composed predominantly of mannose. Because of the close similarity in serologic reactivity between the polysaccharide of *S. telluris* A and the mannan of *C. albicans* A, some structural details of the haptenic determinants of the former are postulated.

References

Ballou, C.E. and William, C.R.: Polymorphism of the somatic antigen of yeast. Science *184:* 127–134 (1974).

Dryer, R.L.; Tammes, A.R., and Routh, J.I.: The determination of phosphorus and phosphatase with N-phenyl-*p*-phenylenediamine. J. biol. Chem. *225:* 177–183 (1957).

Dubois, M.; Giles, A.K.; Hamilton, J.K.; Rebers, P.A., and Smith, F.: Colorimetric method for determination of sugars and related substances. Analyt. Chem. *28:* 350–356 (1956).

Gitlin, D.J.: Use of ultraviolet absorption spectroscopy in the quantitative precipitation reaction. J. Immun. *62:* 437–451 (1949).

Hasenclever, H.F. and Kocan, R.M.: Serotypes in *Saccharomyces telluris*. Their relation to sources of isolation. Infec. Immunity *7:* 610–612 (1973).

Hasenclever, H.F. and Mitchell, W.O.: Antigenic relationships of *Torulopsis glabrata* and seven species of the genus *Candida*. J. Bact. *79:* 677–681 (1960).

Hasenclever, H.F. and Mitchell, W.O.: A study of yeast surface antigens by agglutination inhibition. Sabouraudia *3:* 288–300 (1964).

Johnson, M.J.: Isolation and properties of a pure yeast polypeptidase. J. biol. Chem. *137:* 575–586 (1947).

Peat, S.; Whelan, W.J., and Edwards, T.E.: Polysaccharides of bakers' yeast. 4. Mannan. J. chem. Soc. 29–34 (1961).

Steward, T.S. and Ballou, C.E.: A comparison of yeasts, mannans and phosphomannans by acetolysis. Biochemistry *7:* 1855–1863 (1968).

Summers, D.F.; Grollman, A.P., and Hasenclever, H.F.: Polysaccharide antigens of *Candida* cell wall. J. Immun. *92:* 491–499 (1964).

Sunayama, H.: Studies on the antigenic activities of yeasts. IV. Analysis of the determinant groups of the mannan of *Candida albicans* serotypes A. Jap. J. Microbiol. *14:* 27–39 (1970).

Sunayama, H. and Suzuki, S.: Studies on the antigenic activities of yeasts. V. Effect of alpha-mannosidase digestion on the immunochemical properties of the mannan of the *Saccharomyces cerevisiae.* Jap. J. Microbiol. *14:* 197–207 (1970).

Suzuki, S.; Sunayama, M., and Saito, T.: Studies on the antigenic activities of yeasts. I. Analysis of the determinant groups of the mannan of *Saccharomyces cerevisiae.* Jap. J. Microbiol. *12:* 19–24 (1968).

Yu, R.J.; Bishop, C.T.; Cooper, F.P.; Hasenclever, H.F., and Blank, F.: Structural studies of mannans from *Candida albicans* (serotypes A and B), *Candida parapsilosis, Candida stellatoidea* and *Candida tropicalis.* Can. J. Chem. *45:* 2205–2211 (1967).

Dr. *H.F. Hasenclever,* National Institute of Allergy and Infectious Disease, Rocky Mountain Laboratory, *Hamilton, MT 59840* (USA)

Histoplasma Antigens: Their Production, Purification and Uses[1]

L. Pine

Products Development Branch, Center for Disease Control, Public Health Service, US Department of Health, Education and Welfare, Atlanta, Ga.

Introduction

The early history and evolution of our knowledge of histoplasmosis is excellently described in Histoplasmosis (*Sweany*, 1960). The two national conferences on histoplasmosis (U.S. Dept. HEW, 1956; *Ajello et al.*, 1971) supply a complete spectrum of references which bring us up to the last several years of research on the antigenic nature of the fungus *Histoplasma capsulatum*. The purpose of this review is to integrate earlier and more recent results concerning the overall antigenic composition of the yeast and mycelial phases of the fungus; to describe specific antigens; and to emphasize certain aspects relating to the production and application of these antigens. The importance of histoplasmosis in the United States alone has recently been emphasized by *Ajello* (1971), *Larsh* (1971) and *Campbell* (1974). An estimated 200,000 cases of acute pulmonary infection and 70 deaths occur yearly, with an estimated infection rate of 40 million persons (*Furcolow*, 1969). These statistics make histoplasmosis, with little question, the most important of the deep mycoses when number of deaths per year, man-hours lost and cost are considered. This has been evidenced in the Biological Products Division, Center for Disease Control (CDC) Atlanta, Georgia by a marked increase in demand for *Histoplasma* serological reagents; within the last 5 years, requests for such products as histoplasmin and yeast phase antigen have more than doubled. The original *Histoplasma* antigens were the culture filtrate (histoplasmin) of the mycelial phase and formolized yeast. These were used as skin test antigens or complement-fixing antigens (*Tenenberg*, 1960).

---

[1] This review is written in memory of Dr. *Arden Howell, jr.*, a friend with whom I collaborated in much of my research and a major contributor to our knowledge of histoplasmosis.

Since then, there has been a constant search for products which would give a greater degree of sensitivity and specificity in the serological diagnosis of the disease (*Cross and Howell,* 1948; *Kaufman,* 1971; *Larsh,* 1971). *Howell* (1947) distinguished the parameters which had to be considered in evaluating histoplasmin to be used for the skin test and defined a critical titer for evaluating heterologous activity in *Blastomyces*-infected animals. *Howell* emphasized that lots of antigen vary greatly and that evaluation of the antigen depends upon methods of comparing the size of the skin test reaction with the level of sensitivity of the animals used.

The complexities of antigen production must be considered within the scope of *Howell*'s observations because a reliable and specific quantitative assay for the antigen is essential to the production of any given microbial antigen. Then, the methods to be used for animal sensitization or for production of the serum required for antigen evaluation must be considered. Live-cell infection of an animal, hyper-sensitization with killed cells with or without adjuvant, the methods of killing cells or of making cell derivatives, the route of inoculation, the species of animal used, and the serological test itself are factors that may have a direct and specific relationship to the product which will be isolated. Thus, agar gel precipitin, capillary tube precipitin, complement fixation, reactivity with fluorescent antibody, hemagglutination and skin test reactivity may deal with separate antigenic substances, and therefore dual or multiple activities cannot be attributed to a given antigen until it is highly purified.

Once the quantitative test has been evaluated and decided upon, the production of the antigen itself entails consideration of fermentation parameters and processes such as autolysis, feed back controls, induction, repression, or strain variation. Finally, assuming that biochemical purification is relatively straightforward and that it is productive, we should recognize that the final purified antigen may not have the all-encompassing desirable characteristics we observed in the original crude product.

Growth and Maintenance of Histoplasma *Mycelial and Yeast Phases*

Howell (1939) performed a morphological study of the development of microconidia, macroconidia and cellular forms of *H. capsulatum* and compared it to that of similar species. The "life cycle" and physiology of *Histoplasma* have been reviewed by *Pine* (1960) and *Bauman* (1971). The sexual stage, *Emmonsiella capsulata,* was discovered and described by *Kwon-Chung* (1972, 1973); it is obtained by growing the heterothallic mating strains in Alphacel-yeast-extract agar, yeast-extract agar or soil-extract agar. For stock cultures, both *Pine* (1970) and *Berliner* (1971) have emphasized that yeast phase is best for preserving the characteristics of a given strain. The yeast phase will maintain the sporulating characteristics of the mycelial phase and will demonstrate these characteristics when converted at 25° C.

Generally, the mycelial phase is maintained on Sabouraud's agar slants at 25° C, although transfers on such media rapidly result in the loss of sporulating ability and subsequent conversion to a white, essentially sterile variant (*Pine, 1960*). *Berliner* (1971) has classified two of the many different mycelial variants as A (albino with smooth macroconidia) and B (brown with tuberculate spores); *Tewari and Berkhout* (1972) have shown that type B is more pathogenic for mice than type A. In general, passage of nonsporulating variants through animals will not change the sporulating characteristics of the fungus (*Pine, 1970; Berliner, 1971*), although variation may occur by passage through the animal (*O'Hern, 1964*). Physiological and morphological variation occurs rapidly by transfer of the mycelial strain in Sabouraud's or similar media; once lost, the original characteristics appear extremely difficult, if not impossible, to regain.

Pine (1970) has described a mycelial maintenance medium which maintained the cultural and morphological characteristics of six strains over 20 years. This medium is best prepared with 1.5% agar and slanted in screw-cap tubes. After the slant is inoculated, the cultures should be incubated for approximately 1 month at 25° C with the screw cap sufficiently loose to permit free passage of air. When stored at 4° C, such cultures have remained viable for 1 to 3 years. Preparations of this medium are commercially available; they are satisfactory only for the growth and maintenance of the mycelial phase. Although such preparations may be used for growth of the yeast phase by adding citric acid, the autoclaved yeast phase medium which results lacks the growth-supporting and mycelial-to-yeast converting qualities obtained by preparing the medium in two separate halves as described by *Pine* (1970). Certain important details in the preparation of yeast phase and mycelium media are given below.

It is best to maintain stock cultures in the yeast phase if the particular strain can be obtained in this form. The yeast phase conversion and maintenance medium, originally described by *Pine and Drouhet* (1963) is essentially identical to the mycelium medium described above, but contains in addition citric acid, which serves primarily as a chelating agent of Ca and Mg ions to suppress mycelial growth (*Pine and Peacock,* 1958). Alpha ketoglutarate and the citrate also serve as substrates which stimulate the rate of growth and increase the cell yields of the yeast phase. The medium has all the vitamins required for maximum growth reported by *Salvin* (1949), *Pine* (1957) and *McVeigh and Morton* (1965). In addition, the medium contains cysteine (not cystine), which is required not only for the conversion of the mycelial phase to the yeast phase (*Salvin,* 1949; *McVeigh and Houston,* 1972) but also for the maintenance of viability and growth of 10^2 to 10^6 yeast phase cells (*Rowley and Huber,* 1955; *Pine,* 1955). It also contains starch as a binder of oleic acid to which the organism is extremely sensitive but still requires as a growth factor in finite amounts (*Pine,* 1954).

Although considerable evidence has been presented that heavy cell suspensions of the yeast phase are capable of metabolizing cystine with (*Gilbert and Howard,* 1970) or without the presence of an added energy source (*Garrison et al.,* 1970), the overwhelming evidence cited above suggests that cysteine, with an active −SH, is required for growth of small inocula of yeast-phase cells. This finding is further supported by the data of *Garrison et al.* (1970). Of all the low molecular weight compounds which they tested, L−cysteine gave the greatest increase in yeast-phase cell respiration. Further, in simple synthetic media at a pH greater than 6.5, cysteine, in the presence of metallic ions, rapidly converts to cystine, and crystallizes from the medium. When this happened, no growth occurred, even though the medium was saturated with cystine (*Pine,* 1954). The optimal pH 6.5 for growth was also found by *Gilbert and Howard* (1970) to be optimal for cystine uptake. Furthermore, compounds forming loose ionic or covalent structures with the −SH of cysteine inhibit growth (*Pine,* 1954, 1955). That *McVeigh and Morton* (1965) found growth of the yeast phase equally responsive to cysteine or cystine may be explained in part by the fact that in preparing the medium, cystine was solubilized by heating in a strongly alkaline solution. Such a procedure may well lead to the formation of −SH compounds.

We recommend the media of *Pine and Drouhet* (1963); *Pine,* (1970) for maintaining stock cutures of the yeast phase and for use in converting the mycelial phase to the yeast phase; we also recommend the *Pine* medium (1970) for maintenance of the mycelial phase.

Although some might argue that *Pine*'s media are difficult to prepare, no crude medium has been found which gives equal or more satisfactory results for growth and sporulation of the mycelial phase and, with citric acid, for the growth and maintenance of the yeast phase (*Pine,* 1970). No medium which unequivocably surpasses the yeast-phase medium for its ability to convert the mycelial phase to the yeast phase has been found (*Haley and Standard,* 1976). The mycelial phase, when grown to a stage of heavy sporulation, will remain viable for 1 to 3 years when stored at 4° C; the yeast phase, after 7 to 8 days' growth, at which time it should have reached the stationary phase, will remain viable for 1 to 2 years when stored at 4° C. We prefer, however, to transfer the yeast phase at 6-month intervals.

Preparing the medium is simple after the vitamin suspension, minor element solution and other solutions have been made. All solutions are stable and may be stored at 4° C for several years, particularly if care is taken to prevent microbial growth during this period by judiciously adding several drops of chloroform. The growth factors, lipoic acid and coenzyme A, are frozen for storage. All other solutions inhibit microbial growth during storage because of their pH. When the media are slanted in tightly stoppered screw-cap tubes, they are stable for 6 months to a year at 4° C. Screw-cap test tubes are preferred because they prevent rapid evaporation during the long periods of incubation required for growth of the mycelial or yeast phases and for conversion to the yeast phase. But the fungus is strongly aerobic, and if the free passage of air is stopped by the glass expanding at 37° C, growth will cease. The final pH 6.5 is critical, and the media should not be made more alkaline. The formula calls for "insoluble potato starch". For the yeast-phase medium, citric acid, not sodium citrate, is used. The yeast phase is extremely sensitive to free oleic acid, and the yeast phase medium must be regulated for this factor. For this reason, oleic acid and starch are controlled as described in a footnote (*Pine*, 1970) for the preparation of liquid or semisolid agar.

Excellent growth of the yeast phase is also obtained with the synthetic medium of *McVeigh and Morton* (1965). Media which contain added gross organics, which are very simply prepared, and which support good growth of the yeast phase, are the casamino acid medium of *Salvin* (1956) and the brain-heart infusion medium with 1% cysteine (*Berliner*, 1971).

Sabouraud's medium should not be used for maintenance of mycelial phase strains. Based on the results of *Artis and Baum* (1963) and *Anderson and Marcus* (1968), Sabouraud's agar with phosphate might be used for this purpose. The results of the meticulous study by *Yen and Howard* (1970) suggest that the casein hydrolysate medium described or the medium of *Rowley and Huber* (1955) is most suitable for the germination of yeast-phase cells and conversion to mycelium. The latter medium supported 70 to 90% germination of 100 yeast-cell aggregates.

No medium gives an absolute guarantee of converting the mycelium to the yeast phase. In all cases agar slants used for this conversion should have sufficient water of syneresis or added broth to keep the medium moist for several weeks. In this regard, use of 1.25% agar or the addition of 0.5 ml of broth to tubes covered with aluminum caps or loose screw caps is suggested. Three media are strongly recommended: the mycelial phase maintenance medium with citric acid as described above (*Pine*, 1970); the *Kurong Yegian* (1954) inspissated egg medium, and the *Francis*-medium with cystine (*Campbell*, 1947). A piece of mycelial mat approximately 1 cm^2 should be placed on the slant, and macerated to small fragments with a strong inoculating needle. The slant is incubated at 37° C. It should be tilted daily to moisten the agar surface. Conversion may occur within 10 days or may require 1 to 2 months; it may be complete, with only gross or small yeast phase colonies appearing, or, if the mycelial phase grows and covers the surface, petite yeast-phase colonies may form at various places. They can be seen with a hand lens on the agar surface beneath the mycelium. The yeast phase should be isolated from a single colony. Variations within the yeast phase isolates are readily demonstrated when 100 to 200 cells of the yeast phase of stock culture are permitted to convert back to the mycelial phase; in liquid media, colonies having different morphological features are readily observed (*Rowley and Pine*, 1955). If conversion *in vitro* is unsuccessful, mice or hamsters should be inoculated (*O'Hern*, 1964).

Several media and their specific uses have been described above with the emphasis on obtaining and maintaining stock cultures to be used in preparing fungal reagents. Although the subject is outside the scope of this paper, one medium is strongly recommended (*Haley and Standard*, 1976) for primary isolation of the mycelial phase from clinical materials; this is the Sabhi medium (Sabouraud's agar plus brain-heart infusion agar) of *Gorman* (1967).

Antigens of the Yeast Phase

Antigens and Strain Specificity of the Whole Cell

The polymeric nature of the yeast cell surface is such that "the antigenic properties of yeasts can be explained mainly on the basis of the mannan-protein component of the cell wall" (*Ballou and Raschke*, 1974). Common surface antigens may relate widely divergent taxons; on the other hand, specific antigenic differences of the surface antigens may distinguish serotypes within the same well-defined species. Thus *Hasenclever and Mitchell* (1961) described the A and B antigenic types of *Candida albicans*; differentiation of these types rested upon an agglutination reaction with absorbed sera produced by rabbits hyperimmunized with viable or heat-killed cells.

In a study of the variation in complement fixation of different yeast phase strains of *H. capsulatum*, *Schubert and Ajello* (1957) observed a wide range of reactivity of cells killed by Merthiolate[2]. Two strains, 105 and B11, gave little if any, complement fixing reaction with rabbit sera, but B11 was essentially unreactive with human sera. Similar results were obtained in a study of the comparative fluorescein-labeled antibody staining of *H. capsulatum* and *Histoplasma duboisii* with a specific anti-yeast phase *H. capsulatum* conjugate (*Pine et al.*, 1964). Although most of the *H. capsulatum* strains reacted strongly with the specific conjugate, two strains, 6617 and 6621, did not. Neither did any of the *H. duboisii* strains. This was so, regardless of the medium used for growth and regardless of whether the strains were passed into hamsters in which they caused marked infection. Strains 6617 and 6621 showed much higher anthrone reagent-reactive carbohydrate than the other strains of *H. capsulatum* tested; when tested as complement-fixing antigens, these two strains did not react with human sera (*Pine et al.*, 1966). Since the media used for growth were very different, and since inoculation into animals did not induce antigenicity, failure of these strains to produce strong antigenic components did not appear to be related to growth or regulating factors of the medium. Although the comple-

---

[2] The use of trade names is for identification only and does not constitute endorsement by the Public Health Service or by the Department of Health, Education and Welfare.

ment fixation reactivity of some strains is affected quantitatively to a small degree by growth in diverse media, the reactivity of most strains is not changed. Similar results and considerations with diverse media were reported by Markowitz (1967, 1969).

Using fluorescein-labeled antiglobulins obtained from rabbits hyperimmunized with 0.5% formalin-killed yeast phase cells, Kaufman and Blumer (1966) explained the above results when they described four different surface antigens of *Histoplasma* which were capable of delineating five separate serotypes (1,2; 1,4; 1,2,3; 1,2,4; and 1,2,3,4). Serotype 1,4 represent 46% of the cultures studied; all 11 strains of *H. duboisii* and all 5 strains of *Blastomyces dermatitidis* examined were also of this antigenic composition. Strains 6617 and 6621 were the 1,4 serotype (*Kaufman*, personal commun.).

Strains of *H. capsulatum* serotypes 1,2,3 and 1,4 and *H. duboisii* were then examined with regard to their chemical composition (*Pine and Boone*, 1968). Although extracting the unbroken cells of serologically reactive strains did not affect their complement-fixing ability or change their reactivity with heterologous sera (*Pine et al.*, 1966), breakage of the cell released strong complement-fixing antigens closely associated with the insoluble protein-carbohydrate complexes of the 1,2,3 serotype-cells. Crude cell walls of serotype 1,4 still did not react with either the specific fluoresceinated conjugate or, in the complement-fixation test, with human sera (table I). Strains of the 1,2,3 serotype contained only 16–30% sulfuric acid-releasable glucose as compared to the 1,4 serotypes of *H. capsulatum* and *H. duboisii* which contained 63–75% (table II). However, strains of serotype 1,2,3 had greater amounts of protein associated with their cell wall and higher concentrations of chitin, as expressed by their susceptibility to chitinase. In 3% NaOH they showed different solubilities than the 1,4 serotype (table II). Treatment of the serotype 1,2,3 cell walls with pepsin and trypsin did not destroy the ability of the walls to react with unabsorbed fluorescein conjugate or with specific adsorbed anti-*Histoplasma* conjugate (table I), although such treatment consistently increased the relative reactivity of these antigens with human anti-*Histoplasma* sera. Of the sugars observed in a 24-hour hydrolysis of crude cell walls with sulfuric acid, major amounts of glucose, smaller amounts of mannose, small amounts of hexosamine and traces of galactose were found. Uronic acid was not detected. Extraction of crude cell walls with 3% NaOH for 6 hours in a boiling water bath released insoluble polysaccharide from the 1,2,3 serotypes. The polysaccharide was reactive with the specific fluorescein-conjugate and in the complement fixation tests. The insoluble product of the 1,4 serotypes, although reactive in complement fixation tests, did not react with the absorbed fluorescein-globulin (table III). A similar NaOH-insoluble polysaccharide, obtained by pretreatment of trypsin-pepsin digested cell walls of serotypes 1,2,3 with $2\,N\ H_2SO_4$, was shown to have glucose, mannose, galactose and hexosamine. This fraction obtained from the

Table I. Reactivity of whole cells and cell wall preparations of H. capsulatum strains with fluorescein-labeled antiglobulin and in complement fixation tests

Strain	Fluorescein-globulin reaction									Complement fixation[c]					
	live cells			crude cell walls[b]			trypsin-pepsin digested walls			crude cell walls		trypsin digested walls		trypsin-pepsin digested walls	
	NC[a]	CC	AC	NC	CC	AC	NC	CC	AC	H[d]	B[e]	H	B	H	B
H. capsulatum															
F851	±	+5	+2	—	+5	+5	+1	+5	+5	128	64	512	256	512	64
A811	±	+5	+5	±	+5	+4	±	+5	+5	128	64	512	128	512	128
6624	±	+5	+4	±	+5	+5	—	+5	+5	256	128	512	128	512	64
6617	—	+5	—	—	+5	—	—	+5	—	0	64	0	0	0	0
6621	—	+5	±	—	+5	—	—	+5	—	0	64	0	0	0	0
H. duboisii															
828	—	+5	—	+5	+5	+5	—	+5	—	0	64	0	0	0	0
2591	—	+5	—	+5	+5	+5	—	+5	—	0	64	0	0	0	0

[a] NC = normal serum conjugate; CC = crude antiglobulin conjugate; AC = absorbed conjugate.
[b] Cell walls were prepared as indicated in table I, *Pine and Boone* (1968).
[c] Crude cell walls were prepared from washed cells, killed by freezing and thawing. The cells were ruptured sonically and the cell wall residues obtained by centrifugation were dried and stored as acetone powders.
[d] H = anti-*Histoplasma* serum (human).
[e] B = anti-*Blastomyces* serum (rabbits).

Table II. Chemical differentiation of *Histoplasma* serotypes

Reaction of cell walls	*Histoplasma capsulatum*		*Histoplasma duboisii*
	serotype 1, 2, 3 (3 strains)	1, 4 (2 strains)	1, 4 (2 strains)
% dry wt. released by proteinase	52–69	27–28	28–30
% dry wt. released by chitinase	67–80	19–26	not done
% of total protein and carbohydrate released by chitinase	50–92	0–5	not done
% insoluble in 3% NaOH	42–44	21–30	not done
% soluble in 3% NaOH	48–49	62–68	not done
% dry wt. released by $2N\ H_2SO_4$ (24 Hr.):			
Glucose	16–30	63–75	72
Amino acid	3–8	0.5	0.5
Hexosamine	7–8	2–3	3–5

Data from *Pine and Boone* (1968)

Table III. Complement fixation titers of and reaction to anti-*Histoplasma* (fluorescein-tagged conjugates by cell wall fractions of different serotypes extracted with sodium hydroxide.

Strain and serotype[a]	NaOH extracted cell wall residues					NaOH soluble non-dialyzable extract		
	crude[b] Fl. Ab	absorbed Fl. Ab	complement fixation			complement fixation		
			reciprocal of antigen dilution	reciprocal of titer		reciprocal of antigen dilution	reciprocal of titer	
				H[c]	B		H	B
F851 (1,2,3)	+							
		+	128	512	64	8	1024	512
A811 (1,2,3)	+	+	128	512	32	16	256	64
6624 (1,2,3)	+	+	128	512	32	4	1024	256
6617 (1,4)	+	–	16	256	32	8	64	64
6621 (1,4)	+	–	128	256	32	8	128	64

a All strains were tested on the basis of an original concentration of 5 mg (dry wt.)/ml, *Pine and Boone* (1968).
b Fl-Ab = anti-*Histoplasma* fluorescein conjugate
c H = human anti-*H. capsulatum* serum; B = human anti-*B. dermatitidis* serum

serotype 1,4 had only glucose and hexosamine. Although these data do not definitively describe the chemical nature of either the complement-fixing or fluorescein-globulin reactive antigens, they strongly implicate a polysaccharide portion of the antigens. A protein antigen would not be expected to withstand the enzymatic treatment coupled with both strong acid and alkaline hydrolysis at elevated temperatures. On this basis, one can anticipate that the surface antigens of serotype 1,2,3 contain the specified four carbohydrates, whereas those of serotype 1,4 contain only glucose and hexosamine. The results also imply that serotype antigens 2,3 are required to effectively induce complement-fixing antibody in acquired human infections and that the surface-oriented complement fixing antigen is not made effectively by the yeast phase of the 1,4 serotype. Strains 6617 and 6621, however, can make mycelial phase histoplasmin comparable in its complement fixing ability with immune human sera to that histoplasmin produced by strains of 1,2,3 serotype.

On the basis of observations of the reactions of the cell walls of the different serotypes with heating in 3% NaOH, *Pine* (1972) described a simple chemical test which distinguishes the serotypes 1,2,3 and 1,4. Two to three loopfuls of yeast-phase cells are suspended in 5 ml of 1% NaOH and heated in a test tube in a boiling water bath for 10 min. Serotypes 1,4 will give a smooth suspension of cells which is stable for 15 to 30 min; serotypes 1,2,3, however, form a coarse coagulum which rapidly settles to the bottom of the tube.

Domer (1971) isolated cell-wall constituents of the yeast phase by ethylene-diamine extraction of defatted cell walls; without defining serotypes, the chemical analyses confirmed the two distinct groups of *Histoplasma* cell walls as reported by *Pine and Boone* (1968) and confirmed the high content of chitin by direct analyses of N-acetyl glucosamine in the group demonstrating low total monosaccharide. In the chemotype II, 22.8% of the total glucose existed as a glucan which was ethylene-diamine soluble-water insoluble; this fraction was absent from the chemotype I. Similarly, *Anderson et al.,* (1974), using phenol extraction procedures for analyses of two strains, found the components of the cell wall residue to be essentially identical to those reported above for the two groups.

Yeast Phase Antigens Released into the Medium during Growth

The soluble antigens released into the medium during the growth of the yeast phase must be considered from a different aspect than those released from the cell proper. In general, polysaccharides and proteins excreted into the medium are by-products of growth and represent a particular stage of controlled or derepressed metabolism; soluble antigens present in the culture broth may have the same chemical constituents bound to or soluble within the yeast phase cell. Certain of them may be antigens released as a result of autolysis of the yeast phase cell and may be components of the cell. In this sense, the Y antigen of

Tompkins (1965) is considered below as a cellular product, because it is obtained in greater yields by direct extraction of viable cells with phenol.

Sorensen and Evans (1954) precipitated soluble products from the neopeptone broth filtrates of the yeast phase, using Zn acetate. After the Zn was removed by adding phosphate to the soluble antigen, protein was removed by repeated chloroform extraction. The soluble product which remained was fractionated by ethanol precipitation. This product, believed to be a polysaccharide free of protein, was reactive in the complement fixation reaction with anti-*Histoplasma* rabbit serum and did not react with sera of rabbits infected with *B. dermatitidis*. A similar product was obtained by killing neopeptone-grown cultures with 1% phenol or formalin and fractionating the filtered medium (*Dyson and Evans,* 1955). The fractions obtained by 67–75% ethanol were excellent skin-test antigens in animals infected with *Histoplasma*; the antigen was inactivated by repeated chloroform extraction. Essentially, the same method of fractionation was followed by *Knight and Marcus* (1958) in their search for a skin-test antigen which might serve as a primary standard; in this case, the yeast phase was grown with agitation in tryptose phosphate broth containing cysteine. This product, which was much more reactive in *Histoplasma*-infected animals than in those infected with *Blastomyces,* was negative in the biuret test, had no pentose, and contained 4% nitrogen, 1.07% phosphorus and 75–90% reducing sugars including 59% hexose. In skin tests with human volunteers (*Edwards et al.,* 1961) the product compared favorably with histoplasmin. Although the product was considered a polysaccharide, the 0.01 mg used was 100 times more concentrated on the basis of dry weight than the estimated amount of dry substance in the control histoplasmin-lot 42, and small amounts of protein were thought to play a role in the skin test reaction.

Salvin and Smith (1959) purified an antigen which was also a potent skin-test antigen when tested in hypersensitive guinea pigs and in humans; this product also increased the resistance of mice to lethal challenge. It did not, however, react as a complement-fixing antigen. For the first time, the constituent carbohydrates and protein were characterized. The product, isolated from culture filtrates, was obtained primarily by dialysis against various concentrations of ethanol; the fraction containing between 50–75% ethanol was most reactive and specific, being approximately 1,000 times more reactive in the animal sensitized with the homologous antigen than in the animal sensitized with *B. dermatitidis*. Chemical examination showed the product to contain lipid, 1.5 to 4.2% nitrogen and 29–37% glucose. Mannose and trace amounts of galactose and a third unidentified sugar were present. The carbohydrate was associated by strong ionic attraction to a protein showing a complete spectrum of amino acids and having an absorption maximum at 280 nm. Cross reactivity was attributed to the protein moiety. *Markowitz* (1964) described procedures for isolating polysaccharide from culture filtrates. He obtained three major antigens present in the crude material which were reactive in the precipitin and skin tests. Two contained significant amounts of protein; all had at least two antigens. Growth reached its maximum in 5 days; antigens did not appear until 7 days after inoculation and increased up to the twentieth day. Continued study with such antigens strongly suggested that reaction of the antigen with precipitating or complement fixing antibody was related to strain specificity (*Markowitz*, 1967). Chemical analyses of such antigens showed that they were primarily galactomannans or gluco-galactomannans with different molar ratios of the sugars, dependent upon the strain from which they were isolated. Strong reactions of purified antigens with concanavalin A (*Markowitz*, 1969) implied the presence of free C–3, C–4, and C–6 hydroxyls of the terminal glucopyranose or mannopyranose residues of highly branched polysaccharides (*Goldstein and Iyer*, 1966).

Soluble, Insoluble and Cell Wall Antigens Released by
Processing the Yeast Phase Cell

Results of analyses and evaluations of the cell fractions with regard to their chemical composition and antigenicity will reflect in part the method of killing the cell, the method of disrupting the cell and, finally, the source of antibody used to measure the antigenic reactivity of the preparation. In these matters, choices may be approached from either the chemical or the disease standpoint. From the chemical standpoint, the investigator is concerned not only with the gross chemical composition of a macromolecule but also with its stereoconfiguration as related to its activity as an antigen. Antisera so produced can be used to relate the chemical configuration of similar antigens taken from the same organism, and also similarly isolated polymers from among widely different microbial species. Thus *Andrieu et al.* (1969), used soluble antigen, which produced hypersensitization of animals, from culture filtrates of similar species to show taxonomic relations between *H. capsulatum, H. duboisii, H. farciminosum, Gymnoascus demonbreunii, B. dermatitidis* and *Paracoccidioides brasiliensis*. Similarly, *Azuma et al.* (1974) demonstrated that galactomannan isolated from the whole cells of *H. capsulatum* species, *B. dermatitidis,* and *P. brasiliensis* were immunogenic and that the immunological polymer was common among all the species. In both investigations, the immune serum was a diagnostic tool for discriminating or relating compounds which might appear chemically similar, if not identical.

From the other standpoint, the investigator is concerned with antigens related to disease. In this case, the antiserum is viewed as the reagent in the quantitative assay whereby one discriminates one macromolecule from among many being isolated. The assay procedure may be based upon capillary precipitin, agar gel precipitin, complement fixation or skin test reactivity, and it must be assumed that, until proven otherwise, these serological procedures evaluate separate antigens. Separate antigenic sites of the same molecule may, however, be differentially reactive. Thus, antigens reactive in the capillary precipitin test may not be reactive when tested by complement fixation. Nor can it be assumed that immunization of an animal with whole cells or fractions thereof induces antibodies common to those resulting from natural infections (*Bradley et al.*, 1974).

In their fractionation of yeast phase cells reacting with human anti-*Histoplasma* sera in the complement fixation test, *Pine et al.*, (1966) observed a marked difference in breakage of live cells as compared to those killed with pyridine or formalin; when treated with sonic energy, live cells broke rapidly. Furthermore, attention was drawn to the Merthiolate-killed cells, which reacted to sonication as did live cells and which consistently gave more specific reactions than did formalin-treated cells in the complement fixation tests. This observation was further investigated with over 25 homologous and heterologous sera to compare the formalin or Merthiolate-killed antigens of two strains grown on brain-heart infusion agar and on casein hydrolysate cysteine agar. The results showed that treatment of *Histoplasma* yeast-phase cells with formalin consistently increased the reactivity of this antigen with heterologous sera. (*Pine et al.*, 1969). *Reeves* (personal commun.) found that the supernate of the standard thimerosol-killed yeast-phase cells was highly reactive and more specific than was the whole thimerosol-killed suspension. The soluble preparation reacted in only 12.1% of 141 tests with heterologous sera, whereas the whole-cell yeast phase suspension reacted in 47.3% of 91 such tests (*Reeves et al.*, 1972). The reactivities of the two types of antigens with homologous sera were essentially the same. Further examination of the soluble yeast-phase preparation showed that the H and M antigens described by *Heiner* (1958) were present with mixtures of low molecular weight antigens. The mixture was termed Y antigen (*Reeves et al.*, 1974). The Y antigen was highly reactive as a complement-fixing antigen and was specific for antihistoplasmosis sera. Depending upon the particular strain of yeast phase used, the antigens were formed in mixtures of H.M.Y; H.Y plus traces of M; or Y plus traces of H antigen. All partially purified antigens showed the presence of protein and carbohydrate. Of 60 sera examined, 38% reacted with the Y antigen, 32% reacted to purified H antigen, and 77% reacted with the purified M antigen. Of other reagents tested for releasing the soluble antigen from the yeast phase, 0.02% iodoacetate appeared to be the best; formalin again induced strong reactions with heterologous sera. Since the Y antigen complex absorbed at 260 nm and had a low molecular weight, it may have contained the soluble antigen described by *Tompkins* (1965).

Recently, *Feit and Tewari* (1974) described the properties of yeast-phase ribosomes and their effectiveness as immunogens. The ribosomes, which were released by homogenization with glass beads in a Braun homogenizer, were separated on a sucrose gradient and characterized as 77S particles. They were composed of approximately 55% protein and 45% RNA; were free of DNA; had 3–4% or less carbohydrate and a 260/280 absorption ratio of 1.9; and sedimented as a single homogeneous fraction. Immunizing mice with ribosomes gave 80% to 90% of the protection afforded by immunization with 5×10^5 live yeast phase cells, if adjuvant was used with the ribosomes. Treating the ribosomes with ribonuclease or ribunuclease and pronase before using them as immunogens reduced their activity by 85%. Preliminary experiments have shown that the protein fraction of the preparation is the principal factor responsible for the immunogenic response. Serological reactivity of the ribosomal preparation or its protein have not been reported.

Salvin and Ribi (1955) compared the immunogenicity of the cell wall and protoplasmic fractions of Merthiolate-killed or ether-killed yeast cells disrupted with glass beads in a Mickle homogenizer. The reactivity of the antigenic fractions obtained by the two methods was about the same, but the reactivities of the various fractions of the homogenates differed greatly. Cell wall preparations had more complement-fixing activity with human histoplasmosis sera than did the whole unruptured cell, whereas the filtered cell protoplasm was much less reactive than the whole cells. In addition, the cell wall fractions were the best antigens for inducing high-titered complement-fixing antibody in rabbits, in accord with subsequent data of other workers. The chemical composition of the cell wall and the antigenic nature of certain constituents have already been discussed in part.

Comparative Analyses of Yeast and Mycelial Phases

From a NaOH-soluble, acetate-soluble fraction, *Azuma et al.* (1974) have isolated a highly purified galactomannan of the mycelial phase cells of *H. capsulatum* and *H. duboisii*. This product, which was antigenic, was not obtained from the yeast phase cells; however, it reacted strongly with sera from rabbits immunized with heat-killed formalinized yeast phase and showed a strong immunodiffusion band like that produced by a similar antigen obtained from strains of *B. dermatitidis* and *P. brasiliensis* when anti-*H. capsulatum* serum was used. Methylation studies showed that the galactomannans contain a $1 \rightarrow 6$-linked mannopyranoside backbone, with branching at the 3 or 2 position of the main chain.

The presence of $1 \rightarrow 3$ and $1 \rightarrow 2$-linkages was also suggested in the main chain. In skin tests, the antigens produced an Arthus type skin reaction. They also produced the capillary precipitin reaction, and the galactomannan of all species gave a single arc of identity with rabbit anti-*H. capsulatum* serum. Because the mannan of *Alternaria kikuchiana* Tanaka did not react with the anti-*H. capsulatum* serum in the quantitative precipitin test, the investigators suggested that the terminal nonreducing galactofuranosyl residue plays an impor-

Table IV. Chemical comparison of yeast phase and mycelial phase cell wall fractions[a]

Determination	Description	Yeast phase, %[b]	Mycelial phase, %[b]
Cell wall	yeast phase-glucan = 60%α, 40%β-glycoside mycelial phase- 100%β glycoside		
Total phosphorus		0.15	0.34
Hexoses:		81.7	32.4
Glucose		77.5	18.8
Galactose		2.3	7.5
Mannose		5.4	17.2
Amino sugar		11.5	25.8
Amino acids		7.1	12.4
Alkali-soluble, non-precipitable fraction	(galactomman + glycoprotein)		
Yield		3.3	22.7
Total phosphorus		0.64	0.67
Hexoses		20.7	24.0
Yeast phase[c]	glu: gal: man = 1.0:1.4:1.4		
Mycelial phase[c]	gluc: gal: man = 1.0:6.8:13.2		
Amino sugar		1.1	0.8
Amino acids		29.0	28.1
Alkali-soluble, precipitable fraction	α (C1→3)glycoside small amount (1→4) or (1→6)		
Yield		41.7	0.0
Total phosphorus		0.0	—
Total nitrogen		0.02	—
Hexose	glucose only	99.5	
Alkali-insoluble residue	yeast phase-52% β (1→3)glycoside mycelial phase-73% β (1→3)glycoside		
Yield		47.5	64.1
Total phosphorus		0.06	0.09
Hexoses		60.7	30.7
Yeast phase	glu: gal: man = 1.0:0.1:0.1		
Mycelial phase	glu: gal: man = 1.0:0.1:0.2		
Amino sugar		23.0	37.7
Amino acids		11.1	10.1

tant role as an immunological determinant of galactomannans. From these data and the results of *Grappel et al.* (1969), *Azuma et al.* (1974) concluded that two major groups of galactomannans are present as serologically reactive polysaccharides in fungi. One group, having primarily 1 →6-linked D-mannopyroanosyl residues as the main chain, is composed of the genera *Histoplasma, Paracoccidioides, Blastomyces, Candida, Saccharomyces* and some dermatophytes. The second group, having 1→ 2, 1 → 6 linked D-mannopyranosyl residues as the main chain, contains the genera *Aspergillus, Penicillium* and *Cladosporium*.

Several groups of workers (*Kobayashi and Guiliacci*, 1967; *Domer et al.*, 1967; *Kanetsuna et al.*, 1974) have compared the chemical structure of the cell walls of the mycelial and yeast phases. *Kobayashi and Guiliacci* (1967) found that the alkali-resistant material of the mycelium had more protein that did that of the yeast-phase. Amino acid analyses of the alkali-resistant fractions showed only small differences between the two phases; the yeast phase had a low threonine content and apparent low tyrosine and phenylalanine contents as compared to the mycelial phase. *Pine* (1972) attempted to distinguish the yeast and mycelial phases of *H. capsulatum* serotypes 1, 2, 3 from those of *H. capsulatum* and *H. duboisii* serotypes 1,4 by amino acid analyses of cell walls previously digested with trypsin and pepsin. The *H. capsulatum* serotypes 1,2,3 appeared to differ from serotypes 1,4 by having higher lysine, arginine, and threonine contents but a lower combined mole concentration of glycine plus serine. *H. duboisii* 1,4 serotypes differed from those of *H. capsulatum* by having significantly higher threonine contents. The cell walls of the mycelial phases of all serotypes were closely similar in their amino acid composition. *Domer et al.*, (1967) found the yeast phase had more chitin and smaller amounts of mannose and amino acids than the mycelial phase. When treated with chitanase, the cells of the mycelial phase released much larger amounts of associated glucose than the yeast phase. Both glucose and mannose were observed, with the yeast phase having a 7:1 ratio of glucose to mannose in an ethylenediamine-soluble water-soluble fraction. In the mycelial phase this ratio was essentially reversed.

Kanetsuna et al. (1974), in a remarkably thorough study of the polysaccharide composition of the cell walls of the yeast and mycelial phases of a single strain, observed marked differences between the two phases, not only in the quantitative aspects of the polysaccharide present, but qualitative differences of sugar composition and configuration. These results are summarized in table IV.

---

[a] The strain analyzed, (G-184B-Chemotype 11, serotype 1,4?).

[b] Values are percent of the fraction analyses, except for the yield, expressed as percent of the cell wall. Hexoses, amino sugar and amino acids were estimated with glucose (as $C_6H_{10}O_5$), N-acetylglucosamino (as $C_0H_{13}NO_5$) and alanine as standards respectively.

[c] glu = glucose, gal = galactose, man = mannose.

Modified table of *Kanetsuna et al.* (1974).

Particularly noteworthy was the fact that the cell wall of the mycelial phase contained glucans which had only β-glycosidic linkages while the yeast phase had 40% β-glycoside and 60% α-glycoside linkages. With the strain used, hexoses represented approximately 82% of the yeast-phase cell wall, and only 32% of the mycelial phase cell wall. In both phases, glucose was the predominate sugar, although the mycelial phase had proportionately a much higher amount of mannose. In addition, the yeast phase had an alkali-soluble, precipitable fraction, which was 99.5% α(1 →3) glucan with finite amounts of (1 →4)-or (1 →6) linkage. This fraction was absent from the mycelial phase. Glucomannan and glycoprotein were observed in alkali-soluble, non-precipitable fractions; significant amounts of galactose, amino acids, and amino sugars were also constituents of these fractions which were observed as 22.7% of the mycelial phase but only 3.3% of the walls of the yeast phase (table IV). Examination of the composition of the cell wall of the yeast-phase showed a glucose composition of 77.5% with 47.5% as an alkali-insoluble residue. These values suggest a serotype 1,4 strain of *H. capsulatum* (*Pine and Boone,* 1968). *Kanetsuna et al.* (1974) recognized their strain as a chemotype II of *Domer* (1971); on analyzing type 1 by chemical means and electron microscopy, they found no α-glucan or α-glucan fibrils. Thus, chemotype I (serotype 1,2,3) appears to be devoid of the α-glucan; this difference from chemotype II suggested to these workers that separate species designation might be considered.

Antigens of the Mycelial Phase

In the preceding section, the chemical composition of the cell wall of the mycelial phase was described. Although only antigenic characteristics of the galactomannan of *Azuma et al.* (1974) were reported, there is little doubt that other fractions of the cell wall are also antigenic or possess serological reactivity. *Reiss et al.* (1974) have described a galactomannan complex isolated from the whole defatted mycelium of *H. capsulatum*. The complex, which was isolated by extraction with 0.25 *N* NaOH, represented 7.5% of the dry weight of the cells and was nondialyzable. The complex was separated by diethylamino-ethyl-cellulose chromatography into two components, a galactomannan and a glycoprotein, both having a galactose-to-mannose ratio of 2:5. Both products showed a heavy band of identity in immuno-diffusion tests with antiserum from an infected rabbit; the galactomman-protein also contained a second reactive component at a much lower concentration. Both the glycoprotein and the galactomannan inhibited sensitized macrophage migration, although the latter antigen had approximately one-tenth the activity of the glycoprotein. Only the glycoprotein, however, reacted positively as a skin test antigen in guinea pigs immunized with the crude NaOH-extracted complex. Pertinent to its skin test reactivity, the amino acid and sugar composition of the glycoprotein strongly resembles the composition of the purified skin-test antigen isolated by *Bartels* (1971) from lot 42 histoplasmin. Although its sugar and amino acid composition also resembles that of the H and M antigens of *Bradley et al.* (1974), it does not react with human or animal antibody specific for these antigens (*Reiss*, unpublished results).

Kobayashi (1971) isolated a polysaccharide from culture filtrates of the mycelial phase grown for 6 months on glucose-yeast-extract broth. Steps involving dialysis, concentration, treatment with proteolytic enzymes and chromatography on ion-exchange resins ultimately yielded a glucomannan free of ninhydrin-reactive material. The product was reactive in agar immunodiffusion tests with the serum of rabbits immunized with the killed mycelium of *H. capsulatum*; it had a molecular weight of about 20,000 and a sedimentation coefficient of 2.53, as shown by ultracentrifugal studies. Some skewness of the leading edge of the sedimentation pattern suggested minor heterogeneity.

Factors Influencing the Production of Histoplasmin

Since it serves as the basic component in several important diagnostic procedures, the product histoplasmin is probably the most important of the crude antigens formed by *H. capsulatum*. Historically, histoplasmin was prepared by growth of the mycelial phase for several months at room temperature in a modified *Smith*'s asparagine glucose glycerol medium (*Emmons et al.*, 1945). Filtrates obtained in the method served three basic uses. First, they were used as skin-test antigens, once they had been standardized with regard to a critical reactivity which minimized heterologous activity and nonspecific reactions in normal volunteers (*Shaw et al.*, 1950). *Goodman* (1971) recently emphasized that such antigens not only react in skin tests with *B. dermatitidis* and *Coccidioides immitis*-infected animals, as observed earlier (*Emmons et al.*, 1945), but also react with guinea pigs infected with *A. terreus*, *A. fumigatus*, *Sporothrix schenckii*, *Emmonsia crescens*, *Penicillium* species, and *Beauveria* species.

Second, *Tenenberg and Howell* (1948) described a complement fixation reaction using histoplasmin as the antigen. They pointed out that although the antigen reacted with heterologous sera from *B. dermatitidis*- and *C. immitis*-infected animals, it was much more reactive with homologous sera.

Finally, *Heiner* (1958) found that concentrated histoplasmin gave immunodiffusion precipitin lines which were of significant diagnostic importance in evaluating human sera; particularly important were the H and M antigens. *Tompkins* (1965) observed that M precipitin appeared early in some infections and the H-precipitin later; some patients did not seem to develop antibodies to the H antigen. *Kaufman* (1971, 1973) states that, in general, the H-precipitin is found in patients who have active and progressive disease and that this antibody may persist for up to two years after clinical recovery, whereas the M-precipitin is indicative of active infection, a past infection, or recent skin testing. The M-precipitin is a longer lasting antibody than the anti-H antibody.

Although the same product has been used unchanged or in a concentrated form as a reagent for these three serological tests, there is no unequivocable data indicating whether one antigen could react in all three tests. *Salvin and Hottle* (1948) observed that when the *Smith* medium was inoculated with mycelial phase, little skin testing or complement-fixing antigen formation was observed until after two weeks' incubation; titers increased as the carbohydrate sources were used up and as the pH increased. These workers found that filtrates which did not react in the skin-test reaction did not fix complement. Although *Salvin and Hottle* (1948) had recommended glycogen as the preferred substrate for antigen production, *Schubert et al.* (1953) found that *Smith*'s medium (*Emmons et al.*, 1945) was superior; *Schubert et al.* (1953) emphasized strain variation as a cause of variation in the production of complement fixing antigens. Further support of the glucose glycerol asparagine medium as the medium of choice came when *Schubert and Wiggins* (1966) compared it to a medium composed of peptone, meat extract and glucose. These workers also observed that stagnant cultures in which the mycelial matts dropped beneath the liquid surface, or which formed no surface growth, gave either no antigen or poor yields. *Wiggins and Schubert* (1965) made several important observations pertinent to different lots of histoplasmin, the presence of H and M antigens, and reactivity with complement. They found that, in general, only three types of histoplasmin were formed — those with H antigen; with H and M antigens; and those with no H or M antigens. If no H or M antigens were formed, then a negative complement fixation reaction would be obtained. They observed that the formation and identification of the precipitin bands were affected by the concentration of the antigen and the arrangement of the wells containing the antigen and serum. Their data strongly supported the conclusion that the complement fixation titer represented the sum of antibody reactions to the H and M antigens. By using a box titration of antigen and antibody to obtain maximum sensitivity for the formation of precipitin lines, they obtained titers of sera by immunodiffusion which were only two dilutions less than those obtained in the complement fixation test. These workers felt that the H band occurred too infrequently to be used as an effective measure of active disease. Additional complexities of the immunodiffusion test have been described by *Gross et al.* (1975).

In the past, the production of histoplasmin suitable for use in either complement fixation or precipitin tests was based upon choice of the several culture flasks showing good antigen production from among the many which did not. Recently, *Ehrhard and Pine* (1972a, b) investigated and attempted to delineate those factors which would lead to consistent production of satisfactory lots of histoplasmin to be used primarily for the production of H and M antigens, and which could also serve as a complement fixing antigen. The method that evolved was based primarily upon the use of yeast phase as inoculum for growth of mycelial strains known to produce H or H + M antigens. The use of the yeast phase permitted a standard heavy homogeneous inoculum to be prepared; subsequent cultures incubated at 25° C, with or without shaking, invariably showed constant characteristics among all the flasks and gave consistent and predictable yields of antigen. Little difference was observed among three synthetic or semisynthetic media tested for the production of histoplasmin; since the *Smith*-asparagine medium was simpler to make, it was preferred. Of prime importance was the choice of the correct strain, since strains not only varied as to the type and amount of antigen produced but also in the rapidity which they converted to an antigen-forming mycelium. Changes in the basic composition of the asparagine medium did not increase the yields of antigens or induce the differential formation of one antigen over the other; glucose was required for good antigen production. The results showed that both H and M antigens were released during growth and during the stationary phase; M antigen was also shown to be a product of autolysis.

Very recently, *Standard and Kaufman* (1976) developed an extremely novel and specific immunological test for the rapid identification of members of the genus *Histoplasma*. On the basis of evidence that the H and M antigens are specific for *Histoplasma* (*Kaufman and Clark*, 1974; *Bauman and Smith*, 1975), these workers developed a rapid procedure for the analyses of H or H + M antigens produced in brain-heart infusion broth by species of *Histoplasma*; identification of these antigens with specific antisera in the immunodiffusion test permitted rapid identification of nonsporulating strains or similar morphological forms without conversion to the yeast phase *in vitro* or *in vivo*.

Purification of Skin-Test Antigen of H. capsulatum.

Cross and Howell (1948) precipitated a skin-test-reactive polysaccharide from a lot H–14 histoplasmin by using a low pH to remove protein and repeated alcohol precipitation for purification. The product was found free of protein by several tests, and reducing sugars were demonstrated after hydrolysis. This product was reactive in the skin test with guinea pigs infected with *H. capsulatum*, showed very low cross reactivity with animals infected with *B. dermatitidis*, and was approximately 10 times more reactive than the original histoplasmin on a mg weight basis.

The most significant progress in delineating the nature of the skin-test antigens of histoplasmin was that reported by *Bartels* (1971), who used standard skin-test antigen Lot–42. Using disc electrophoresis to evaluate the number of components and to identify those which were reactive in the skin test, *Bartels*, in preliminary tests, found five protein fractions, two of which also showed a positive *Schiff*-base reaction for polysaccharides. These two glycoproteins were the only products which gave a positive skin test reaction; they had Rf values relating to the frontal buffer of 0.38 and 0.7 respectively. After using acrylamide gel preparative electrophoresis for isolation, *Bartels* found that the two active components contained glucose, galactose, mannose and hexosamine. In the product with an Rf value of 0.7 there was a complete spectrum of amino acids, of which proline, glutamic acid, aspartic acid, threonine, serine, glycine and alanine were present in this order of higher to lower molar concentrations. Tyrosine, phenylalanine, histidine were present in lowest concentrations. End-group analysis indicated that histidine was the N-terminal amino acid, whereas both serine and threonine were the carboxyl terminal groups. Based primarily on evidence from electrophoretic mobility and amino acid composition tests, the skin test antigens were found to bear a strong resemblance to the H and M antigens partially purified later by *Bradley et al.* (1974).

Purification of H and M Antigens of Histoplasmin

Greene et al. (1960) and, still later, *Dickerson and Busey* (1968) reported the separation of H and M antigens of histoplasmin using diethylaminoethylcellulose with a decreasing pH and increasing salt molarity gradient in phosphate buffer. M antigens appeared in fractions of pH 6.1 to 8, whereas H antigen appeared in fractions of pH 5.5 to 5.1. Although there was a major concentration of H or M antigen, other workers did not find these antigens separated from one another with the lots of histoplasmin tested (*Wiggins and Schubert*, 1965). Based upon these results, *Bradley et al.* (1974) used several additional procedures of purification and stepwise elution from diethylaminoethylcellulose of increasing acidity by addition of $0.1\,M$ tris (hydroxymethyl)aminomethane. Fractions of H and M antigen were obtained which appeared to be about 9–12% contaminated with other products. However, the two antigens reacted only with sera from proven or suspect cases of histoplamosis and showed reactivity with those sera known to contain only the anti-H or anti-M antibody, respectively. No reaction was observed with heterologous sera; agar immunodiffusion tests indicated no H antigen present in the M antigen, and *vice versa,* with 26 histoplasmosis sera used. The H antigen reacted with one of eight blastomycosis sera. Both antigens were found to be glycoproteins containing glucose, galactose and mannose in a ratio of 1:1:2.3 for the M protein and an average 1:7.5:14 for two H antigens. The relative amino acid composition was nearly the same as that reported by *Bartels* (1971) for the skin test antigen. In the case of the M antigen, proline, threonine, glutamic acid and serine appeared to have higher concentrations than those observed in H antigen. The antigens both appeared to be ionic complexes of one to four protein-containing substances with a range of molecular weights from 25,500 M_r for an apparent single antigen to greater than 200,000 M_r for the complex. Treatment of the purified antigens with lysozyme, snail-gut chitinase, trypsin or chymotrypsin did not implicate either the carbohydrate or the protein portion as antigenic sites; although the purified antigens were readily

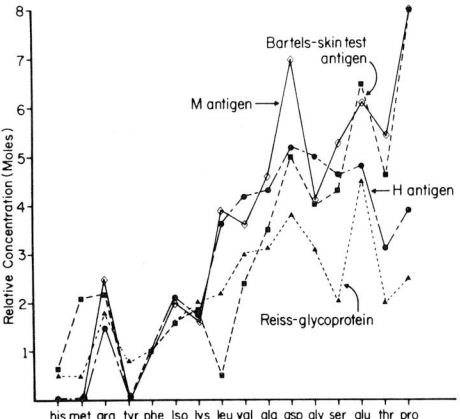

Fig. 1. Comparative amino acid composition of *Histoplasma* skin-test reactive antigens and highly purified H and M antigens of histoplasmin. Data from *Bartels* (1971), *Reiss et al.* (1974) and *Pine, Gross, Bradley and Moss,* unpublished data).

inactivated by placing them for 10 minutes in a boiling water bath, none of the enzymatic treatments caused a loss of reactivity in agar gel double-diffusion tests.

Later examination of all purified M antigens showed a secondary antigenic component termed "non-M" (*Green and Harrell,* unpublished results); when concentrated sufficiently, all purified H antigens showed traces of M antigen. The H and M antigens were freed of these contaminants by performing a second chromatographic step using diethylaminoethylcellulose and stepwise decrease in the pH of 0.1 M phosphate buffer from 7.4 to 4.0 (*Pine, Gross, Bradley and Moss,* unpublished results). The individual purified H and M antigens were then passed into preparative acrylamide gel slabs by electrophoresis from which they were isolated as single discrete bands. The carbohydrate-to-protein ratios of the H and M antigens were 1:2.1 and 1:0.8, respectively; the maximum absorption was at 268 to 270 nm; and the 260/280 absorption ratios were 1.023 to 1.080. The amino acid composition of each was essentially the same as that reported for the 25,000 M_r-M antigen and the 34,000 M_r-H antigen, respectively (*Bradley et al.,* 1974). Figure 1 shows the comparative relationship of *Reiss'* skin test galactomann with the highly purified H antigen and that of *Bartels'* glycoprotein to M antigen. Depending upon the serological test, the antigens gave strong reactions when 2–16 µg were used. The two highly purified antigens reacted only with homologous H or M antibody from immunized rabbits or with 137 human anti-histoplasmosis sera in agar gel immunodiffusion and complement fixation tests. In complement fixation tests with 37 heterologous sera, one human serum from a proven case of blastomycosis showed a 1:32 titer with the M antigen and a 1:2 titer with the H antigen; another serum reacted with the M at a titer of 1:4. Preliminary tests in guinea pigs sensitized with *H. capsulatum* showed that they were highly positive at 0.5 μg protein as skin test antigens and elicited no reaction in normal animals (*Selin and Pine,* unpublished results). *Sprouse* (1971) has shown that two glycoproteins, isolated from histoplasmin by electrophoresis on acrylamide gels, elicited delayed hypersensitivity in *Histoplasma*-infected guinea pigs at 0.05 and 0.06 μg. One fraction, d II, had a molecular weight of less than 300,000 M_r and appeared homogeneous by electrophoretic and sedimentation tests. The overall results strongly support the conclusion that the H and M antigens of *Heiner* are reactive as precipitating antigens in the capillary precipitin and agar immunodiffusion tests, as complement fixing antigens, and as skin-test antigens.

Purified Histoplasma *Antigens — Their Value and Uses*

The antigens of both the yeast and mycelial phases are described in tables V and VI. Microbiologists and biochemists prefer to deal with the pure antigen itself. There is little doubt that antigenic, serological, and chemical conclusions based upon studies with the pure substance eliminate the ambiguous, if not erroneous, conclusions drawn from studies of a product that is not pure. Unquestionably, studies with pure products give a much deeper and fundamental basis for understanding the source of the antigen, its chemical nature and its mode of reaction.

There are relatively few advantages to be gained from the use of pure products in general serological procedures. Thus, one may require a primary standard reference product for use as a skin-test reagent (*Knight and Marcus,* 1958; *Shaw et al.,* 1950) or a product which, when used as an immunogen, is free from secondary undesirable effects. The results of *Kaufman et al.* (1969) indicate that a single skin test with the M antigen may elevate the complement fixation titer. These workers suggest "that the use of a skin-test antigen purified to contain only H component would detect histoplasmin hypersensitivity without inducing antibodies and would eliminate false-positive serological reactions caused by the M component.". From the serological standpoint, one requires specificity and sensitivity, but it is also evident from the serological evaluations of *Kaufman* (1973) that diagnosis of histoplasmosis rests upon a thorough use and evaluation of several procedures. Each could ultimately require a battery of purified reagents, no one of which might have the chemical stability or the antigenic range of reactivity exhibited by a "well balanced" crude complex.

The application of *Histoplasma* antigens covers a wide range. Yeast-phase whole antigens demonstrate specific serotypes with fluorescein-labeled specific antibody. They are used to examine for the yeast phase in clinical materials. The

Table V. Antigens of *H. capsulatum*-yeast phase

	Source	Serological activity	Composition	Reference
1	Surface antigen	serotyping reaction with fluorescein-tagged globulin	galactose-trace, hexosamine galactomannan glucan	*Pine and Boone* (1968) *Domer* (1971)
2	Excreted soluble	complement fixation	polysaccharide	*Sorensen and Evans* (1954)
3	Excreted soluble	skin-test	polysaccharide	*Dyson and Evans* (1955)
4	Excreted soluble	skin-test	polysaccharide	*Knight and Marcus* (1958)
5	Excreted soluble	skin-test immunizing	glycoprotein glucomannan-protein-complex trace galactose	*Salvin and Smith* (1959)
6	Excreted soluble	precipitin skin-test	glycoprotein-complex galactomannan gluco-galactomannan precipitated by concanavalin A	*Markowitz* (1969)
7	Excreted	precipitin	undefined	*Andrieu et al.* (1969)
8	Whole cell, extracted with phenol	precipitin	5000 MW, 260 absorption, 4% P, 15% N	*Tompkins* (1965)
9	Soluble, released by thimersol and iodoacetate	complement fixation precipitin	small molecular weight-protein complex, large molecular weight glycoproteins H and M antigens	*Reeves et al.* (1972) *Reeves et al.* (1974)
10	Ribosomes	immunizing	77S ribosome-protein complex	*Feit and Tewari* (1974)
11	Cell fractions cell wall	complement fixation		*Salvin and Ribi* (1955)
12	Cell fractions cell wall	complement fixation	carbohydrate-protein complexes	*Pine et al.* (1966)

Table VI. Antigens of *H. capsulatum* - mycelial phase

Source	Serological activity	Composition	Reference
1 Excreted-soluble (histoplasmin)	skin-test	polysaccharide	*Cross and Howell* (1948)
2 Excreted-soluble grown in glucose yeast extract broth	precipitating antigen with rabbit anti-mycelial phase sera	glucomannan molecular weight = 20,000 M_r sed. coef. = 2.53	*Kobayashi* (1971)
3 Excreted-soluble (histoplasmin)	skin-test	glycoprotein, glucose, galactose, mannose, two complexes, electrophoretic Rf- 0.38 and 0.70, high concentration of proline, glutamic, aspartic acids. Tyrosine, phenylalanine, histidine lowest in concentration Histidine = N-terminal, serine and threonine = COOH terminal	*Bartels* (1971)
4 Excreted-soluble (histoplasmin)	capillary precipitin agar gel immunodiffusion, complement fixing, skin-test	glycoprotein, glucose, galactose, mannose, hexosamine, *Heiner*'s H and M antigens. M antigen-higher in proline, threonine and glutamic acid than H antigen. Histidine, tyrosine, methionine low or absent	*Bradley et al.* (1974) *Pine et al.* (unpublished data)
5 Whole cell NaOH extract	skin-test precipitating antigen with antirabbit sera; macrophage inhibition	galactomannan, protein galactomannan, amino acids similar to those above. Glutamic acid in highest concentration; tyrosine, methionine and histidine in lowest concentrations	*Reiss et al.* (1974)
6 Cell wall	capillary precipitin agar gel immunodiffusion	galactomannan (1 →6) linked mannopyranoside, branching at 2 and 3 carbon.	*Azuma et al.* (1974)

yeast phase also releases soluble H and M precipitating antigens and an important complex of Y antigens required for the complement fixation test. The mycelial phase releases soluble H and M antigens and other products used in the agar gel immunodiffusion, complement fixation, capillary precipitin and skin tests. Highly purified products may be satisfactory skin test reagents or they may also serve as primary standards for relating one lot of antigen to another. Purified antigens must be used to define the reactivities of lots of sera which may themselves be used as primary standards or standards for comparisons; they have already been used to produce highly reactive and specific rabbit anti-H antigen and anti-M antigen serum (*Green and Harrell,* unpublished results). The importance of H and M antigens is emphasized by *Kaufman and Clark*'s (1974) recognition that the agar immunodiffusion tests are specific for histoplasmosis. *Bauman and Smith* (1975) support this conclusion and emphasize the reliability and simplicity of the immunodiffusion tests when compared to the complement fixation reaction. The data of *Wiggins and Schubert* (1965), *Kleger and Kaufman,* (1973), *Bauman and Smith* (1975) and our own results with the highly purifed H and M antigens support the conclusion that not only are these two antigens specific, but when correctly used in the agar immunodiffusion test, they are essentially as sensitive for titration of antibody levels of human sera as the complement fixation test. For this, purified antigen could well be used as a standard to support the diagnostic evaluation which employs a crude histoplasmin.

References

Ajello, L.: The medical mycological iceberg. HSMHA Hlth Rep. *86:* 437–448 (1971).
Ajello, L.; Chick, E. W., and Furcolow, M.L.: Histoplasmosis. Proc. 2nd National Conference (Thomas, Springfield 1971).
Anderson, K.L. and Marcus, S.: Sporulation characteristics of *Histoplasma capsulatum.* Mycopath. Mycol. appl. *36:* 179–187 (1968).
Anderson, K.L.; Wheat, R.W.; Conant, N.F., and Clingenpeel, W.C.: Composition of cell wall and other fractions of the autolyzed yeast form of *Histoplasma capsulatum.* Mycopath. Mycol. appl. *54:* 439–451 (1974).
Andrieu, S.; Biguet, J.; Dujardin, L. et Vaucelle, T.: Etude antigenique des agents des mycoses profondes par l'analyse comparee des milieux de culture. I. *Histoplasma capsulatum* et *H. duboisii.* Relations avec *H. farciminosum, Gymnoascus demonbreunii, Blastomyces dermatitidis* et *Paracoccidioides brasiliensis.* Mycopath. Mycol. appl. *39:* 97–108 (1969).
Artis, D. and Baum, G.L.: Tuberculate spore formation by thirty-two strains of *Histoplasma capsulatum.* Mycopath. Mycol. appl. *31:* 29–35 (1963).
Azuma, I.; Kanetsuna, F.; Tanaka, Y.; Yamamura, Y., and Carbonell, L.M.: Chemical and immunological properties of galactomannans obtained from *Histoplasma duboisii, Histoplasma capsulatum, Paracoccidioides brasiliensis* and *Blastomyces dermatitidis.* Mycopath. Mycol. appl. *54:* 111–125 (1974).

Ballou, C. and Raschke, W.: Polymorphism of the somatic antigen of yeast. Science *184:* 127–134 (1974).
Bartels, P.A.: Partial chemical characterization of histoplasmin H–42; in Ajello, Chick and Furcolow Histoplasmosis. Proc. 2nd National Conference, pp. 56–63 (Thomas, Springfield 1971).
Bauman, D.S.: Physiology of *Histoplasma capsulatum;* in Ajello, Chick and Furcolow Histoplasmosis. Proc. 2nd National Conference, pp. 78–84 (Thomas, Springfield 1971).
Bauman, D.S. and Smith, Coy D.: Comparison of immunodiffusion and complement fixation tests in the diagnosis of histoplasmosis. J. clin. Microbiology *2:* 77–80 (1975).
Berliner, M.D.: Biological implications of morphological variants in *Histoplasma capsulatum* primary isolates; in Ajello, Chick and Furcolow Histoplasmosis. Proc. 2nd National Conference, pp. 21–29 (Thomas, Springfield 1971).
Bradley, G.; Pine, L.; Reeves, M.W., and Moss, C.W.: Purification, composition, and serological characterization of histoplasmin H and M antigen. Infec. Immunity *9:* 870–880 (1974).
Campbell, C.: Reverting *Histoplasma capsulatum* to the yeast phase. J. Bact. *54:* 263–264 (1947).
Campbell, C.: Respiratory mycotic infection. Prevent. Med. *3:* 517–528 (1974).
Cross, F.C. and Howell, A., jr.: Studies of fungus antigens. II. Preliminary report on the isolation of an immunologically active polysaccharide from histoplasmin. Publ. Hlth Rep. *63:* 169–183 (1948).
Dickerson, W.H., jr. and Busey, J.F.: Chromatographic separation of h and m antigens from histoplasmin. Proc. Soc. exp. Biol. Med. *128:* 654–658 (1968).
Domer, J.E.: Monosaccharide and chitin content of cell walls of *Histoplasma capsulatum* and *Blastomyces dermatitidis.* J. Bact. *107:* 870–877 (1971).
Domer, J.E.; Hamilton, J.G., and Harkin, J.C.: Comparative study of the cell walls of the yeastlike and mycelial phases of *Histoplasma capsulatum.* J. Bact. *94:* 466–474 (1967).
Dyson, J.E., jr. and Evans, E.E.: Delayed hypersensitivity in experimental fungus infections. The skin reactivity of antigens from the yeast phase of *Histoplasma capsulatum.* J. Lab. clin. Med. *45:* 449–454 (1955).
Edwards, P.Q.; Knight, R.A., and Marcus, S.: Skin sensitivity of human beings to *Histoplasma capsulatum* and *Blastomyces dermatitidis* polysaccharide antigens. Amer. Rev. resp. Dis. *83:* 528–534 (1961).
Emmons, C.W.; Olson, B.J., and Eldridge, W.W.: Studies of the role of fungi in pulmonary disease. I. Cross reactions of histoplasmin. Publ. Hlth Rep. *60:* 1383–1394 (1945).
Ehrhard, H.-B. and Pine, L.: Factors influencing the production of H and M antigens by *Histoplasma capsulatum.* Development and evaluation of a shake culture procedure. Appl. Microbiol. *23:* 236–249 (1972a).
Ehrhard, H.-B. and Pine, L.: Factors influencing the production of H and M antigens by *Histoplasma capsulatum.* Effect of physical factors and composition of medium. Appl. Microbiol. *23:* 250–261 (1972b).
Feit, C. and Tewari, R.P.: Immunogenicity of ribosomal preparations from yeast cells of *Histoplasma capsulatum.* Infec. Immunity *10:* 1091–1097 (1974).
Furcolow, M.L.: U.S. National Communicable Disease Center: Mycoses Surveillance, N. 1. April (1969).
Garrison, R.G.; Dodd, H.T., and Hamilton, J.W.: The uptake of low molecular weight sulfur-containing compounds by *Histoplasma capsulatum* and related fungi. Mycopath. Mycol. appl. *40:* 171–180 (1970).
Gilbert, B.E. and Howard, D.H.: Uptake of cystine by the yeast phase of *Histoplasma capsulatum.* Infec. Immunity *2:* 139–144 (1970).

Goldstein, I.J. and Iyer, R.N.: Interaction of concanavalin A, a phytohemagglutinin, with model substrates. Biochim. biophys. Acta *121:* 197–200 (1966).

Goodman, N.L.: Cross reactivity in histoplasmin skin testing; in *Ajello, Chick and Furcolow* Histoplasmosis. Proc. 2nd National Conference, pp. 313–320 (Thomas, Springfield 1971).

Gorman, J.: Sabhi, a new culture medium for pathogenic fungi. Am. J. med. Technol. *33:* 151–157 (1967).

Grappel, S.F.; Blank, F., and Bishop, C.T.: Immunological studies of dermatophytes. IV. Chemical structures and serological reactivities of polysaccharides from *Microsporum praecox, Trichophyton ferrugineum, Tricophyton sabouraudii* and *Trichophyton tonsurans.* J. Bact. *97:* 23–26 (1969).

Greene, C.H.; DeLalla, L.S., and Tompkins, V.N.: Separation of specific antigens of *Histoplasma capsulatum* by ion-exchange chromatography. Proc. Soc. exp. Biol. Med. *105:* 140–141 (1960).

Gross, H.; Bradley, G.; Pine, L.; Gray, S.; Green, J.H., and Harrell, W.K.: Evaluation of histoplasmin for presence of H and M antigens: some difficulties encountered in the production and evaluation of a product suitable for the immunodiffusion test. J. clin. Microbiol. *1:* 330–334 (1975).

Haley, L.D. and Standard, P.G.: Laboratory methods in medical mycology. (US Dept. of Health, Education and Welfare, PHS, Washington 1976).

Hasenclever, H.F. and Mitchell, W.O.: Antigenic studies of *Candida.* 1. Observation of two antigenic groups in *Candida albicans.* J. Bact. *82:* 570–573 (1961).

Heiner, D.C.: Diagnosis of histoplasmosis using precipitin reactions in agar gel. Pediatrics *22:* 616–627 (1958).

Howell, A., jr.: Studies on *Histoplasma capsulatum* and similar form species. I. Morphology and development. Mycologia *31:* 191–216 (1939).

Howell, A.: Studies of fungus antigens. I. Quantitative studies of cross-reactions between histoplasmin and blastomycin in guinea pigs. Publ. Hlth Rep. *62:* 631–651 (1947).

Kanetsuna, F.; Carbonell, L.M.; Gil, F., and Azuma, I.: Chemical and ultrastructural studies on the cell walls of the yeastlike and mycelial forms of *Histoplasma capsulatum.* Mycopath. Mycol. appl. *54:* 1–13 (1974).

Kaufman, L.: Serological tests for histoplasmosis; their use and interpretation; in *Ajello, Chick and Furcolow* Histoplasmosis. Proc. 2nd National Conference, pp. 321–326 (Thomas, Springfield 1971).

Kaufman, L.: Value of immunodiffusion tests in the diagnosis of systemic mycotic diseases. Ann. clin. Lab. Sci. *3:* 141–145 (1973).

Kaufman, L. and Blumer, S.: Occurrence of serotypes among *Histoplasma capsulatum* strains. J. Bact. *91:* 1434–1439 (1966).

Kaufman, L. and Clark, M.J.: Value of the concomitant use of complement fixation and immunodiffusion tests in the diagnosis of coccidioidomycosis. Appl. Microbiol. *28:* 641–643 (1974).

Kaufman, L.; McLaughlin, D., and Terry, R.T.: Immunological studies with an M-deficient histoplasmin skin-test antigen. Appl. Microbiol. *18:* 307–309 (1969).

Kleger, B. and Kaufman, L.: Detection and identification of diagnostic *Histoplasma capsulatum* precipitates by counterelectrophoresis. Appl. Microbiol. *26:* 231–238 (1973).

Knight, R.A. and Marcus, S.: Polysaccharide skin test antigens derived from *Histoplasma capsulatum* and *Blastomyces dermatitidis.* Amer. Rev. Tuberc. pulmon. Dis. *77:* 983–989 (1958).

Kobayashi, G.S.: Isolation and characterization of polysaccharide of *Histoplasma capsulatum;* in *Ajello, Chick and Furcolow* Histoplasmosis. Proc. 2nd National Conference, pp. 38–44 (Thomas, Springfield 1971).

Kobayashi, G. and Guiliacci, P.: Cell wall studies of *Histoplasma capsulatum*. Sabouraudia *5:* 180–188 (1967).

Kwon-Chung, K.J.: *Emmonsiella capsulata.* Perfect state of *Histoplasma capsulatum.* Science *177:* 368–369 (1972).

Kwon-Chung, K.J.: Studies on *Emmonsiella capsulata.* I. Heterothallism and development of the ascocarp. Mycologia *65:* 109–121 (1973).

Kurong, J.M. and Yegian, D.: Medium for maintenance and conversion of *Histoplasma capsulatum* to yeast phase. Am. J. clin. Path. *24:* 505–508 (1954).

Larsh, H.W.: The public health importance of histoplasmosis; in *Ajello, Chick and Furcolow* Histoplasmosis. Proc. 2nd National Conference, p. 9–17 (Thomas, Springfield 1971).

Markowitz, H.: Polysaccharide antigens for *Histoplasma capsulatum.* Proc. Soc. exp. Biol Med. *115:* 697–700 (1964).

Markowitz, H.: Antibodies in histoplasmosis. J. Bact. *93:* 40–46 (1967).

Markowitz, H.: Interaction of concanavalin with polysaccharides of *Histoplasma capsulatum.* J. Immun. *103:* 308–318 (1969).

McVeigh, I. and Houston, W.E.: Factors affecting mycelial to yeast phase conversion and growth of the yeast phase of *Histoplasma capsulatum.* Mycopath. Mycol. appl. *47:* 135–151 (1972).

McVeigh, I. and Morton, D.: Nutritional studies of *Histoplasma capsulatum.* Mycopath. Mycol. appl. *25:* 294–309 (1965).

O'Hern, E.M.: Studies on histoplasmosis. I. Comparative virulence of variant and parent strain. *Histoplasma capsulatum* in hamsters. Mycopath. Mycol. appl. *22:* 126–174 (1964).

Pine, L.: Studies on the growth of *Histoplasma capsulatum.* I. Growth of the yeast in liquid media. J. Bact. *68:* 671–679 (1954).

Pine, L.: Reaction of fumaric acid with cysteine. J. Am. chem. Soc. *77:* 3153 (1955).

Pine, L.: Studies on the growth of *Histoplasma capsulatum.* III. Effect of thiamin and other vitamins on the growth of the yeast and mycelial phases of *Histoplasma capsulatum.* J. Bact. *74:* 239–245 (1957).

Pine, L.: Morphological and physiological characteristics of *Histoplasma capsulatum;* in *Sweany* Histoplasmosis, pp. 40–76 (Thomas, Springfield 1960).

Pine, L.: Growth of *Histoplasma capsulatum.* VI. Maintenance of the mycelial phase. Appl. Microbiol. *19:* 413–420 (1970).

Pine, L.: Growth on amino acids, cell wall proteins, and hydrolysis of yeast-phase cell wall of *Histoplasma capsulatum* and *H. duboisii.* Sabouraudia *10:* 244–255 (1972).

Pine, L. and Boone, C.J.: Relationship of cell wall composition to serological reactivity of *Histoplasma capsulatum* serotypes and related species. J. Bact. *96:* 789–798 (1968).

Pine, L.; Boone, C.J., and McLaughlin, D.: Antigenic properties of the cell wall and other fractions of the yeast form of *Histoplasma capsulatum.* J. Bact. *91:* 2158–2168 (1966).

Pine, L. et Drouhet, E.: Sur l'obtention et la conservation de la phase levure d'*Histoplasma capsulatum* et d'*H. duboisii,* en milieu chimiquement defini. Annls. Inst. Pasteur, Paris *105:* 798–804 (1963).

Pine, L.; Falcone, R.G., and Boone, C.J.: Effect of thimerosal on the whole yeast phase antigen of *Histoplasma capsulatum.* Mycopath. Mycol. appl. *37:* 1–14 (1969).

Pine, L.; Kaufman, L., and Boone, C.J.: Comparative fluorescent antibody staining of *Histoplasma capsulatum* and *Histoplasma duboisii* with a specific anti-yeast phase *H. capsulatum* conjugate. Mycopath. Mycol. appl. *24:* 315–326 (1964).

Pine, L. and Peacock, C.L.: Studies on the growth of *Histoplasma capsulatum.* IV. Factors influencing conversion of the mycelial phase to the yeast phase. J. Bact. *75:* 167–174 (1958).

Reeves, M.; Pine, L., and Bradley, G.: Characterization and evaluation of a soluble antigen complex prepared from the yeast phase of *Histoplasma capsulatum.* Infec. Immunity *9:* 1033–1044 (1974).

Reeves, M.W.; Pine, L.; Kaufman, L., and McLaughlin, D.: Isolation of a new soluble antigen from the yeast phase of *Histoplasma capsulatum* Appl. Microbiol. *24:* 841–843 (1972).

Reiss, E.; Mitchell, W.O.; Stone, S.H., and Hasenclever, H.F.: Cellular immune activity of a galactomannan-protein complex from mycelia of *Histoplasma capsulatum.* Infec. Immunity *10:* 802–809 (1974).

Rowley, D.A. and Huber, M.: Pathogenesis of experimental histoplasmosis in mice. I. Measurement of infecting dosages of the yeast phase of *Histoplasma capsulatum.* J. infect. Dis. *96:* 174–183 (1955).

Rowley, D.A. and Pine, L.: Some nutritional factors influencing growth of yeast cells of *Histoplasma capsulatum* to mycelial colonies. J. Bact. *69:* 695–700 (1955).

Salvin, S.B.: Cysteine and related compounds in the growth of the yeastlike phase of *Histoplasma capsulatum.* J. infec. Dis. *84:* 275–283 (1949).

Salvin, S.B.: Growth of *Histoplasma capsulatum* in liquid medium. Proc. Conf. on Histoplasmosis. U.S. Department of Health, Education and Welfare. Public Health Monograph No. 39, p. 61 (1956).

Salvin, S.B. and Hottle, G.A.: Factors influencing histoplasmin formation. J. Bact. *56:* 541–546 (1948).

Salvin, S.B. and Ribi, E.: Antigens from yeast phase of *Histoplasma capsulatum.* II. Immunologic properties of protoplasm vs. cell walls. Proc. Soc. exp. Biol. Med. *90:* 287–294 (1955).

Salvin, S.B. and Smith, R.F.: Antigens from the yeast phase of *Histoplasma capsulatum.* III. Isolation, properties, and activity of a protein-carbohydrate complex. J. infect. Dis. *105:* 45–53 (1959).

Schubert, J.H. and Ajello, L.: Variations in complement fixation antigenicity of different yeast-phase. strains of *Histoplasma capsulatum.* J. Lab. clin. Med. *50:* 304–307 (1957).

Schubert, J.H.; Ajello, L.; Stanford, S., and Grant, V.O.: Variation on complement fixation antigen production by different strains of *Histoplasma capsulatum* grown on two media. J. Lab. clin. Med. *41:* 91–97 (1953).

Schubert, J.H. and Wiggins, G.L.: Additional studies of histoplasmin formation. Mycopath. Mycol. appl. *30:* 81–91 (1966).

Shaw, L.W.; Howell, A., jr., and Weiss, E.W.: Biological assay of lots of histoplasmin and the selection of a new working lot. Publ. Hlth Rep. *65:* 583–610 (1950).

Sorensen, L.J. and Evans, E.E.: Antigenic fractions specific for *Histoplasma capsulatum* in the complement fixation reaction. Proc. Soc. exp. Biol. Med. *87:* 339–341 (1954).

Sprouse, R.F.: Preparation and standardization of histoplasmin; in *Ajello, Chick and Furcolow* Histoplasmosis. Proc. 2nd National Conference, pp. 284–293 (Thomas, Springfield 1971).

Standard, P.G. and Kaufman, L.: A specific immunological test for the rapid identification of members of the genus *Histoplasma.* J. clin. Microbiol. *3:* 191–199 (1976).

Sweany, H.C.: Histoplasmosis (Thomas, Springfield 1960).

Tenenberg, D.J.: The serology of histoplasmosis; in *Sweany* Histoplasmosis, pp. 168–188 (Thomas, Springfield 1960).

Tenenberg, D.J. and Howell, A., jr.: A complement fixation test for histoplasmosis. I. Technic and preliminary results on animal sera. Publ. Hlth Rep. *63:* 163–168 (1948).

Tewari, R.P. and Berkhout, F.J.: Comparative pathogenicity of albino and brown types of mice for *Histoplasma capsulatum.* J. infect. Dis. *125:* 504–508 (1972).

Tompkins, V.N.: Soluble antigenic constituents of yeast-phase *Histoplasma capsulatum.* Am. Rev. resp. Dis., suppl. *92:* pp. 126–133 (1965).

US Department of Health, Education and Welfare: Proc. Conf. on Histoplasmosis. Public Health Monograph No. 39 (1956).

Wiggins, G.L. and Schubert, J.H.: Relationship of histoplasmin agar-gel bands and complement fixation titers in histoplasmosis. J. Bact. *89:* 589–596 (1965).

Yen, C.M. and Howard, D.H.: Germination of blastospores of *Histoplasma capsulatum.* Sabouraudia *8:* 242–252 (1970).

Dr. *L. Pine,* Products Development Branch, Center for Disease Control, Public Health Service, U.S. Department of Health, Education and Welfare, *Atlanta, GA 30333* (USA)

Author Index

Abel, R. 48
Abramovici, A. 81
Ajello, L. 2, 7
Aronson, M. 60

Ben-David, A. 1

Chaparas, S.D. 106

Grosse, G. 48

Hasenclever, H.F. 126

Kaplan, W. 20
Kaufman, L. 95
Kletter, Y. 60

Levine, H.B. 106
Louria, D.B. 31

Male, O. 66
McAtee, F.J. 126
Mishra, S.K. 48

Pine, L. 138

Scalarone, G.M. 106
Shahar, A. 60
Staib, F. 48

Subject Index

Abnormal fetal development 81–94
Absidia 11
– corymbifera 11
Acrasiomycetes 8
Acremonium 14
– falciforme 14
– kiliense 14
– recifei 14
Acrotheca 14
– aquaspersa 14
Actinomyces 32
Actinomycetes 2, 24
Adipositas 72
Aflatoxin 82–84, 86, 90, 91
Agaricales 12
Agglutination tests 100
Ajellomyces 11
– dermatitidis 11
Algae 7, 17
Alloxan 42
Amphotericin B 55
Antifungal vaccines, *see* vaccines
Antigenic relationships 26, 121, 126–137
Antigens 106–168
Aphyllophorales 12
Arthroderma 11
– benhamiae 11
– ciferii 12
– flavescens 12
– gertlerii 12
– gloriae 12
– insingulare 12
– lenticularum 12

– quadrifidum 12
– simii 12
– uncinatum 12
– vanbreuseghemii 12
Ascomycetes 7, 13, 17
Ascomycotina 9–11, 13, 17
Aspergillosis 2, 4, 42, 104
– experimental 42
– immunodiagnosis 95, 96
Aspergillus 14, 16, 26, 27, 42, 82, 84, 86, 87, 95, 96, 153
– clavatus 85, 87
– flavus 14, 82, 84, 85, 95
– fumigatus 14, 95, 96, 155
– nidulans 14, 42
– niger 95
– ochraceus 84, 86
– terreus 155
– versicolor 85, 86
Asthma 96

Bacterium pyocyaneum 70, 78
Basidiobolus 11
– haptosporus 11
Basidiomycetes 5, 7, 13, 17
Basidiomycotina 9, 10, 12, 15, 17
Bats 5
BCG 37
Beauvarie bassiana 2
Beauveria 155
Bird embryo 90, 91
Birds 5, 10, 49
Blastomyces 14, 139, 148, 153

Subject Index

- dermatitidis 3, 5, 11, 14, 24, 26, 31, 42, 97, 98, 113, 136, 146, 148, 155
Blastomycetes 10, 13, 15
Blastomycosis 3, 4, 97, 101, 104, 158, 159
- experimental 42
- immunodiagnosis 97
Brettanomyces 66
Bryophyta 7

Cancer 1
Candida 13, 14, 16, 23, 24, 26, 27, 31–39, 47, 66, 67, 74, 76, 77, 99, 105, 153
- albicans 3, 5, 13, 26–28, 30, 32–39, 42, 47, 66, 99, 126–137, 143
- guilliermondii 11, 13, 66
- krusei 11, 13, 66
- parapsilosis 11, 66
- pseudotropicalis 11, 13
- stellatoidea 32, 34, 38, 66
- toxin, see canditoxin
- tropicalis 13, 32, 34, 38, 66
Candidosis 2, 3, 37, 38, 66–78, 104, 105
- experimental 32–39
- immunodiagnosis 99, 100
- mucocutaneous 66–80
Canditoxin 38
Carcinogenic 82, 83
Carcinoma 70, 71, 75, 96
CEP, see counterelectrophoresis
CF, see complement-fixation test
Chick embryo 83–87, 90, 91
Chickens 86, 88, 91
Chlorophyceae 7
Chrysosporium 14, 16
- parvum 14
- – var. crescens 14
Chytridiomycetes 8
Cinematography 60–65
Cladosporium 14, 16, 153
- carrionii 14
- trichoides 14
Classification 7–19
Claviceps purpurea 84, 87
Coccidioides 14
- immitis 3, 5, 14, 26–28, 31, 39, 97, 98, 106–125, 155
- –, preparation of antigen and vaccines 106–125
Coccidioidin 97, 98, 107, 111, 112
Coccidioidomycosis 4, 5, 40, 96, 104, 112

- epidemiology 112
- experimental 40
- immunodiagnosis 97–99
Cochliobolus 11
- spicifer 11
Coelomycetes 10, 15, 17
Complement-fixation test 96–99, 101, 102
Conidiobolus 11
- coronata 11
- incongruus 11
Coprinaceae 12
Coprinus 12
- cinereus 10, 12
Counterelectrophoresis 98, 100, 101
Cryptococcaceae 13, 66
Cryptococcosis 4, 98, 104
- experimental 40, 41, 48–59
- immunodiagnosis 100
- pathogenesis 48–59
Cryptococcus 13, 16, 40, 41
- neoformans 4, 5, 12, 13, 15, 24, 26, 27, 31, 39, 40, 41, 48–59, 60–65, 100
Cunninghamella 11
- elegans 11
Curvularia 14, 16
- geniculata 14
- lunata 14
- senegalensis 14
Cushing's disease 70
Cyclophosphamide 39
Cytostatics 72

Dactylaria 14, 16
- gallopava 14
Dematiaceae 13
Dermatophytes 17
Dermatophytosis 72, 74
Deuteromycetes 13, 17
Deuteromycotina 10, 13–15, 17
Diabetes 42, 70, 72, 74, 75, 88, 89, 91
Diagnosis 20–30
- biological investigations 23, 28
- collecting and submission of specimens 20–22
- cultural examination 20, 26–28
- direct microscopic examination 20, 23–27
- histological examination 23–27
- immunodiagnostic tests 20. 29, 95–105, 127, 128

- physiological tests 28
- processing of specimens 20, 22, 23
Discomycetes 9
Dogs 42
Drechslera 14, 16
- hawaiiensis 16
- speciciferum 16
Ducklings 86

Electron microscopy 60-65
Embryotoxicity 81-94
Emmonsia crescens 155
Emmonsiella 12
- capsulatum 12
Endomyces 11
- candidus 11
Endomycetaceae 11
Endomycetales 11
Entomophthoraceae 11
Entomophthorales 10, 11
Epidemiology of mycoses 2-6, 112, 113, 138
Epidermophyton 14
- floccosum 14
Ergot 81, 87, 88, 92
Ergotoxin 81, 84, 87, 88, 92
Eumycota 8, 10
Eurotiales 11
Exophiala 14
- salmonis 14
- werneckii 14
Experimental mycoses 31-47, 48-59, 82-91, 107-112, 115-121, 148, 154, 155, 157, 158

FA, see fluorescent antibody test
Favus 2
Filobasidiaceae 12
Filobasidiella 12
- neoformans 12, 13
Fluorescent antibody test 22, 23, 25-27, 30
Fonsecaea 14
- compactum 14
  pedrosoi 14
Freund's adjuvant 39, 116
Fusarenon X 85, 88, 90
Fusarium 14, 16, 81, 85, 88
- culmorum 85
- graminearum 85

- nivale 85
- oxysporum 14
- solani 14
- tricinctum 85

Gasteromycetes 10
Geotrichum 14, 16
- candidum 11, 14
Guinea pigs 34, 37, 41, 111, 115-121, 148, 154, 155, 157, 158
Guizotia abyssinica 54
Gymnoascaceae 11
Gymnoascus demonbreunii 149

Hamsters 83, 84, 87, 91
Heart valves 38
Hemiascomycetes 9, 11
Hendersonula 17
- toruloidea 17
Histoplasma 14, 16, 28, 39, 40, 102, 138-168
- antigens-growth and maintenance of mycelial and yeast phases 139-143
- - of the mycelial phase 154, 155
- - - yeast phase 143-154
- - production, purification and uses 138-168
- capsulatum 3, 5, 12, 14, 19, 21-23, 26-28, 30, 31, 39, 40, 101, 102, 106-125, 138-168
- - preparation of antigen and vaccines 106-125, 138-168
- - var. duboisii 14, 19, 26, 32, 102, 143, 144, 146, 149, 151, 153
- farciminosum 14, 102, 149
Histoplasmin 98, 112-121, 136-168
- factors influencing its production 155-157
- purification of H and M antigens 158-160
- - of skin-test antigen 157, 158
Histoplasmosis 4, 5, 39, 40, 97, 98, 104, 112, 138, 158, 160
- epidemiology 4, 5, 112, 113, 138
- experimental 39, 40
- immunodiagnosis 101, 102
Holobasidiomycetidae 12
Horses 81
Hymenomycetes 10, 12
Hyphochytridiomycetes 8

Subject Index

Hyphomyces destruens 10
Hyphomycetes 14–16

ID, see immunodiffusion test 238
IFA, see indirect fluorescent antibody test
Immunodiffusion test 95–102, 105
Immunology, its value for diagnosis and prognosis 95–105
Immunopathies 70, 71
Imperfect fungi 12, 13, 15, 17
Indirect fluorescent antibody test 26, 27, 100

Kloeckera 66
Kluyveromyces 11
– fragiles 11
Kojic acid 84, 87
Kraurosis 74, 75

LA, see latex particle agglutination test
Labyrinthulales 8
Latex particle agglutination test 98–100, 102, 105
Leukocytic rings 60–65
Levamisole 38
Listeria monocytogenes 39
Listeriosis 39
Loboa 14
– loboi 14
Loculoascomycetes 9, 11
Loderomyces 11
– elongosporus 11
Lysergic acid 84, 87, 88

Madurella 14
– grisea 14
– mycetomi 14
Malformation 81–94
Mammals 10, 49
Mastigomycotina 8, 10
McVeigh and Morton synthetic medium 114
Medically important infectious fungi 7–19
Melanconiales 13, 15
Mice 32–47, 48–59, 83–88, 107–110, 112, 148
Microascaceae 11
Microsporum 12, 16
– amazonicum 12, 14
– audouinii 14
– boullardii 14

– canis 12, 14
– cookei 12, 14
– distortum 14
– equinum 14
– ferrugineum 14
– fulvum 12, 14
– gypseum 12, 14
– nanum 12, 14
– persicolor 12, 14
– praecox 14
– racemosum 12, 14
– ripariae 14
– vanbreuseghemii 12, 14
Millipore membrane filter 28
Moniliaceae 13
Moniliales 13, 17
Monkeys 42, 43, 107
Morbidity and mortality 3, 4
Mortierella 11
– wolfii 11
Mucocutaneous mycoses 66–80
Mucor 11, 42
– pusillus 11
– ramosissimus 11
Mucoraceae 11
Mucorales 10, 11
Mucormycosis, see zygomycosis
Mycelia sterila 13, 15
Mycophenolic acid 84, 86, 87
Mycotoxicosis 81–94
Mycotoxins 31, 38, 81–94
Myriangiales 11
Myxomycetes 8
Myxomycota

Nannizzia 12
– borellii 12
– cajetanii 12
– fulva 12
– grubyia 12
– gypsea 12
– incurvata 12
– obtusa 12
– otae 12
– persicolor 12
– racemosa 12
Neotestudina 11
– rosatii 11
Nocardia 22, 24
– asteroides 25, 32

Subject Index

- brasiliensis 25
- caviae 25

Ochratoxins 84, 86, 90
Oomycetes 9, 10
Opportunistic fungi 3, 17, 27, 29, 67, 68, 70
Organ transplantation 1

Paracoccidioides 14, 153
- brasiliensis 3, 5, 14, 26, 32, 149
Paracoccidioidia 112
Paracoccidioidomycosis 97
Pathogenesis of mucocutaneous mycoses 66–80
Patulin 85, 87, 90
Penicillium 14, 16, 84, 86, 97, 153, 155
- brevi-compactum 84, 86
- marneffei 14
- patulum 85, 87
- purpurogenum 85, 86
- rubrum 85, 86
- stoloniferum 84, 86
Peronosporales 10
Petriellidium 11
- boydii 11
Phaeohyphomycosis 4
Phagocytosis 32–35, 37, 39, 41, 42, 52, 56, 60–65
Phialophora 14, 16
- gougerotii 14
- jeanselmi 14
- mutabilis 14
- parasitica 14
- richardsiae 14
- spicifera 14
- verrucosa 14
Phoma 17
- hibernica 17
Phycomycetes 7, 31
Phycomycosis, see zygomycosis
Pichia 11
- guilliermondii 11
- kudriavzevii 11
Piedraia 11
- hortae 11
Pigeons 5, 126
Pigs 84, 85, 88
Pityrosporum 13
- furfur 13

- pachydermatis 13
Plant kingdom 7
Plasmodiophoromycetes 8
Plectomycetes 9, 11
Pleosporaceae 11
Pleosporales 11
Predisposing factors for infections 70
Prototheca 15
- wickerhamii 15
- zopfii 15
Protothecosis 26
Pseudosaccharomycetales 13, 15
Pteridophyta 7
Pyrenochaeta 17
- romeroi 17
- unguis-hominis 17
Pyrenomycetes 9
Pythiaceae 10
Pythium 10

Rabbits 32, 34, 35, 38, 42, 43, 60, 127, 145, 148, 151, 154, 155, 159
Rats 83–91
Reagents for serodiagnosis 104
Rhinosporidium 15
- seeberi 15, 24
Rhizopus 11
- arrhizus 11
- microsporus 11
- oryzae 11, 42
- rhizopodiformis 11, 42
Rhodophyceae 7
Rodents 88
Rubratoxin B 85, 86, 90

Saccardinulaceae 11
Saccharomyces 153
- cerevisiae 126–137
- telluris 126–137
Saccharomycetaceae 11
Safety precautions 28
Saksenaceae 11
Saksenaea 11
- vasiformis 11
Salamander 85, 87, 90
Sarcoidosis 96
Scanning electron microscopy 60–65
Schizomycetes 7
Schizophyllaceae 12
Schizophyllum 12

– commune 12, 13
Serodiagnosis 95–105
Serodiagnostic reagents 104
Serotypes 126–137
Sex hormones 69, 70
Skin tests 97, 102, 111–113, 115–122, 138–168
Spermatophyta 7
Sphaeropsidales 13, 15, 17
Spherule vaccine 106–110
Spherulin 97, 111–113, 118, 121, 122
Sporothrix 15, 16
– schenckii 15, 26, 30, 32, 43, 155
Sporotrichosis 43
– experimental 43
Staphylococcus 36, 37, 74
– aurens 70
Sterigmatocystin 82, 85, 86
Steroids 4, 34, 42, 69, 70, 72, 78
Stilbaceae 15
Streptococcus 74
Streptomyces achromogenes 85, 88
Streptozotocin 85, 88, 89, 91
Swine 84, 85, 88
Syphilis 3
Systemic mycoses, morbidity and mortality 3, 4
Systemic mycoses in modern medicine 2–6

T2 toxin 85, 88, 90
TA, see tube agglutination test
Taxonomy 7–19
Teliomycetes 9, 12
Teratology 81–94
Testudinaceae 11
Thallophyta 7, 8
Torula 15, 16
– dermatitidis 15
Torulopsis 13, 16, 66
– albicans 66
– glabrata 13, 32, 66, 76, 99
– inconspicua 66
– minor 66
Toxins, see mycotoxins
Transfer factor 37, 38, 47, 112
Trichomonas vaginalis 70
Trichomoniasis 76
Trichomycetes 9
Trichophyton 15, 16
– ajelloi 12, 15
– concentricum 15

– equinum 15
– flavescens 12, 15
– gallinae 15
– georgiae 12, 15
– gloriae 12, 15
– gourvilii 15
– longifusus 15
– megninii 15
– mentagrophytes 12, 15
– – var. erinacei 15
– – – interdigitale 15
– – – mentagrophytes 15
– – – nodulare 15
– – – quinckeanum 15
– phaseoliforme 15
– rubrum 15, 70, 73
– schoenleinii 15
– simii 12, 15
– soudanense 15
– terrestre 12, 15
– tonsurans 15
– vanbreuseghmeii 12, 15
– violaceum 15
– yaoundei 15
Trichosporon 13, 16, 66
– cutaneum 13, 73
Trichothecenes 85, 88, 90, 91
Trigonopsis 66
Tube agglutination test 100
– precipitin test 98
Tuberculariaceae 13
Tuberculosis 3, 39, 96
Turkeys 88

Ustilaginales 12
Ustilomaydis 13

Vaccine administration 110
– preparation 106–125
Vaccines 3, 6, 39, 40, 106–125
– experimental studies 39, 40, 108, 110

Zearalenone 85, 88, 90
Zopfia 11
– senegalensis 11
– tompkinsii 11
Zopfiaceae 11
Zygomycetes 9–11, 31
Zygomycosin experimental 42–43
Zygomycosis 4, 42
Zygomycotina 9–11